CrossFit®

LEVEL 1 TRAINING GUIDE

THIRD EDITION

The CrossFit Level 1 Training Guide is a collection of CrossFit Journal articles written since 2002 primarily by CrossFit, Inc. Founder Coach Greg Glassman on the foundational movements and methodology of CrossFit, Inc.

This guide is designed to be used in conjunction with the Level 1 Course to develop the participant's knowledge and trainer skills and as an essential resource for anyone who is interested in improving their own health and fitness.

Some edits to the original articles have been made for the Training Guide to flow as a stand-alone reference, to provide context for readers, and to stay current with the course format. All original works are preserved in the CrossFit Journal.

No seminar other than the CrossFit Level 1 Certificate Course, as run by CrossFit, grants you the title CrossFit Trainer. Official events can only be verified by using CrossFit.com for registration or by emailing seminars@crossfit.com with your inquiry.

Official qualifications for any individual can be verified in CrossFit's Trainer Directory.

Only CrossFit, Inc. offers the CrossFit Level 1 Certificate Course, and the course has no prerequisites. Only successful completion of this course allows a trainer to apply for affiliation with CrossFit. If an affiliate or other fitness organization claims otherwise, it should be reported at crossfit.com/iptheft.

Third Edition
ISBN: 978-0-9986150-7-3
LCCN: 2017941775

METHODOLOGY

MOVEMENTS

TRAINER GUIDANCE

MOVEMENT GUIDE

INDEX

UNDERSTANDING CROSSFIT

Originally published in April 2007.

The aims, prescription, methodology, implementation, and adaptations of Cross-Fit are collectively and individually unique, defining of CrossFit, and instrumental in our program's successes in diverse applications.

AIMS

From the beginning, the aim of CrossFit has been to forge a broad, general, and inclusive fitness. We sought to build a program that would best prepare trainees for any physical contingency—prepare them not only for the unknown but for the unknowable. Looking at all sport and physical tasks collectively, we asked what physical skills and adaptations would most universally lend themselves to performance advantage. Capacity culled from the intersection of all sports demands would quite logically lend itself well to all sport. In sum, our specialty is not specializing.

PRESCRIPTION

CrossFit is: "constantly varied, high-intensity functional movement." This is our prescription. Functional movements are universal motor recruitment patterns; they are performed in a wave of contraction from core to extremity; and they are compound movements—i.e., they are multi-joint. They are natural, effective, and efficient locomotors of body and external objects. But no aspect of functional movements is more important than their capacity to move large loads over long distances, and to do so quickly. Collectively, these three attributes (load, distance, and speed) uniquely qualify functional movements for the production of high power. Intensity is defined exactly as power, and intensity is the independent variable most commonly associated with maximizing the rate of return of favorable adaptation to exercise. Recognizing that the breadth and depth of a program's stimulus will determine the breadth and depth of the adaptation it elicits, our prescription of functionality and intensity is constantly varied. We believe that preparation for random physical challenges—i.e., unknown and unknowable events—is at odds with fixed, predictable, and routine regimens.

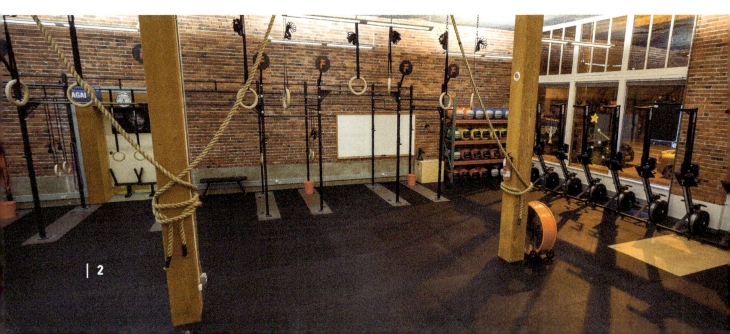

METHODOLOGY

The methodology that drives CrossFit is entirely empirical. We believe that meaningful statements about safety, efficacy, and efficiency, the three most important and interdependent facets to evaluate any fitness program, can be supported only by measurable, observable, repeatable data. We call this approach "evidence-based fitness." CrossFit's methodology depends on full disclosure of methods, results, and criticisms, and we have employed the internet to support these values. Our charter is open source, making co-developers out of participating coaches, athletes, and trainers through a spontaneous and collaborative online community. CrossFit is empirically driven, clinically tested, and community developed.

IMPLEMENTATION

In implementation, CrossFit is, quite simply, a sport—the Sport of Fitness. We have learned that harnessing the natural camaraderie, competition, and fun of sport or game yields an intensity that cannot be matched by other means. The late Col. Jeff Cooper observed that "the fear of sporting failure is worse than the fear of death." It is our observation that men will die for points. Using whiteboards as scoreboards, keeping accurate scores and records, running a clock, and precisely defining the rules and standards for performance, we not only motivate unprecedented output but derive both relative and absolute metrics at every workout; this data has important value well beyond motivation.

ADAPTATIONS

Our commitment to evidence-based fitness, publicly posting performance data, co-developing our program in collaboration with other coaches, and our open-source charter in general have well positioned us to garner important lessons from our program—to learn precisely and accurately, that is, about the adaptations elicited by CrossFit programming. What we have discovered is that CrossFit increases work capacity across broad time and modal domains (see "What Is Fitness? (Part 2)" article). This is a discovery of great import and has come to motivate our programming and refocus our efforts. This far-reaching increase in work capacity supports our initially stated aims of building a broad, general, and inclusive fitness program. It also explains the wide variety of sport demands met by CrossFit, as evidenced by our deep penetration among diverse sports and endeavors. We have come to see increased work capacity as the Holy Grail of performance improvement and all other common metrics like VO_2 max, lactate threshold, body composition, and even strength and flexibility as being correlates—derivatives, even. We would not trade improvements in any other fitness metric for a decrease in work capacity.

CONCLUSIONS

The modest start of publicly posting our daily workouts on the internet beginning in 2001 has evolved into a community where human performance is measured and publicly recorded against multiple, diverse, and fixed workloads. CrossFit is an open-source engine where inputs from any quarter can be publicly given

We've taken high-intensity, constantly varied functional workouts and distilled load, range of motion, exercise, power, work, line of action, flexibility, speed, and all pertinent metabolics to a single value—usually time. This is the Sport of Fitness. We're best at it."

–COACH GLASSMAN

to demonstrate fitness and fitness programming, and where coaches, trainers, and athletes can collectively advance the art and science of optimizing human performance. ■

FOUNDATIONS

Originally published in April 2002.

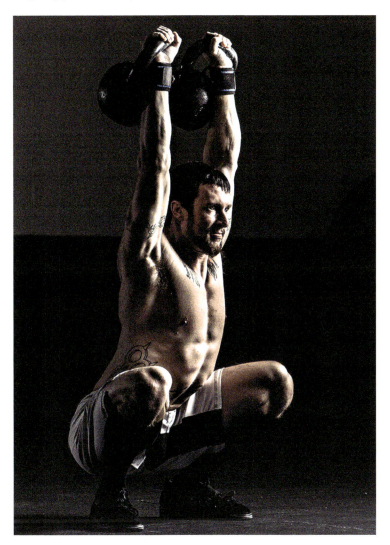

CrossFit is a core strength and conditioning program. We have designed our program to elicit as broad an adaptational response as possible. CrossFit is not a specialized fitness program but a deliberate attempt to optimize physical competence in each of 10 fitness domains. They are cardiovascular/respiratory endurance, stamina, strength, flexibility, power, speed, coordination, agility, balance, and accuracy.

CrossFit was developed to enhance an individual's competency at all physical tasks. Our athletes are trained to perform successfully at multiple, diverse, and randomized physical challenges. This fitness is demanded of military and police personnel, firefighters, and many sports requiring total or complete physical prowess. CrossFit has proven effective in these arenas.

Aside from the breadth or totality of fitness CrossFit seeks, our program is distinctive, if not unique, in its focus on maximizing neuroendocrine response, developing power, cross-training with multiple training modalities, constant training and practice with functional movements, and the development of successful diet strategies.

Our athletes are trained to bike, run, swim, and row at short, middle, and long distances, guaranteeing exposure and competency in each of the three main metabolic pathways.

We train our athletes in gymnastics from rudimentary to advanced movements, garnering great capacity at controlling the body both dynamically and statically while maximizing strength-to-weight ratio and flexibility. We also place a heavy emphasis on Olympic weightlifting, having seen this sport's unique ability to develop an athlete's explosive power, control of external objects, and mastery of critical motor recruitment patterns. And finally we encourage and assist our athletes to explore a variety of sports as a vehicle to express and apply their fitness.

AN EFFECTIVE APPROACH

In gyms and health clubs throughout the world the typical workout consists of isolation movements and extended aerobic sessions. The fitness community from trainers to the magazines has the exercising public believing that lateral raises, curls, leg extensions, sit-ups and the like combined with 20- to 40-minute stints on the stationary bike or treadmill are going to lead to some kind of great fitness. Well, at CrossFit we work exclusively with compound movements and shorter high-intensity cardiovascular sessions. We have replaced the lateral raise with the push press, the curl with the pull-up, and the leg extension with the squat. For every long-distance effort our athletes will do five or six at short distance. Why? Because functional movements and high intensity are radically more effective at eliciting nearly any desired fitness result. Startlingly, this is not a matter of opinion but solid, irrefutable scientific fact, and yet the marginally effective old ways persist and are nearly universal. Our approach is consistent with what is practiced in elite

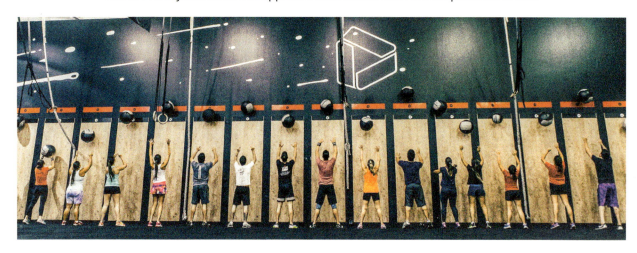

training programs associated with major university athletic teams and professional sports. CrossFit endeavors to bring state-of-the-art coaching techniques to the general public and athlete.

IS THIS FOR ME?

Absolutely! Your needs and the Olympic athlete's differ by degree not kind. Increased power, speed, strength, cardiovascular/respiratory endurance, flexibility, stamina, coordination, agility, balance, and accuracy are each important to the world's best athletes and to our grandparents. The amazing truth is that the very same methods that elicit optimal response in the Olympic or professional athlete will optimize the same response in the elderly. Of course, we cannot load your grandmother with the same squatting weight that we would assign an Olympic skier, but they both need to squat. In fact, squatting is essential to maintaining functional independence and improving fitness. Squatting is just one example of a movement that is universally valuable and essential yet rarely taught to any but the most advanced of athletes. This is a tragedy. Through painstakingly thorough coaching and incremental load assignment, CrossFit has been able to teach everyone who can care for himself or herself to perform safely and with maximum efficacy the same movements typically utilized by professional coaches in elite and certainly exclusive environments.

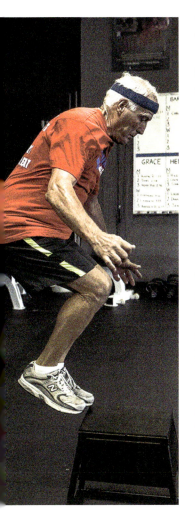

WHO HAS BENEFITED FROM CROSSFIT?

Many professional and elite athletes are participating in CrossFit. Prizefighters, cyclists, surfers, skiers, tennis players, triathletes and others competing at the highest levels are using CrossFit to advance their core strength and conditioning, but that is not all. CrossFit has tested its methods on the sedentary, overweight, pathological, and elderly and found that these special populations met the same success as our stable of athletes. We call this "bracketing." If our program works for Olympic skiers and overweight, sedentary homemakers then it will work for you.

YOUR CURRENT REGIMEN

If your current routine looks somewhat like what we have described as typical of the fitness magazines and gyms, do not despair. Any exercise is better than none, and you have not wasted your time. In fact, the aerobic exercise that you have been doing is an essential foundation to fitness, and the isolation movements have given you some degree of strength. You are in good company; we have found that some of the world's best athletes were sorely lacking in their core strength and conditioning. It is hard to believe, but many elite athletes have achieved international success and are still far from their potential because they have not had the benefit of state-of-the-art coaching methods.

JUST WHAT IS A "CORE STRENGTH AND CONDITIONING" PROGRAM?

CrossFit is a core strength and conditioning program in two distinct senses. First, we are a core strength and conditioning program in the sense that the fitness we develop is foundational to all other athletic needs. This is the same sense in which the university courses required of a particular major are called the "core curriculum." This is the stuff that everyone needs. Second, we are a "core" strength and conditioning program in the literal sense meaning the center of something. Much of our work focuses on the major functional axis of the human body, the extension and flexion of the hips and torso or trunk. The primacy of core strength and conditioning in this sense is supported by the simple observation that powerful hip extension alone is necessary and nearly sufficient for elite athletic performance. That is, our experience has been that no one without the capacity for powerful hip extension enjoys great athletic prowess and nearly everyone we have met with that capacity was a great athlete. Running, jumping, punching, and throwing all originate at the core. At CrossFit we endeavor to develop our athletes from the inside out, from core to extremity, which is, by the way, how good functional movements recruit muscle, from the core to the extremities.

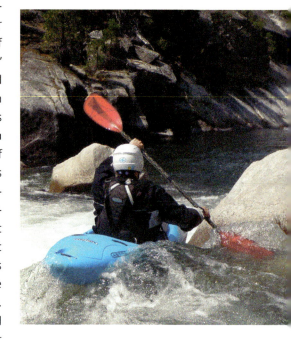

> Significantly improve your 400-meter run, 2,000-meter row, squat, dead, bench, pull-up, and dip. Now you are a more formidable being."
>
> –COACH GLASSMAN

CAN I ENJOY OPTIMAL HEALTH WITHOUT BEING AN ATHLETE?

No! Athletes experience a protection from the ravages of aging and disease that non-athletes never find. For instance, 80-year-old athletes are stronger than non-athletes in their prime at 25 years old. If you think that strength is not important, consider that strength loss is what puts people in nursing homes. Athletes have greater bone density, stronger immune systems, less coronary heart disease, reduced cancer risk, fewer strokes, and less depression than non-athletes.

WHAT IS AN ATHLETE?

According to Merriam Webster's Dictionary, an athlete is "a person who is trained or skilled in exercises, sports, or games requiring physical strength, agility, or stamina."

The CrossFit definition of an athlete is a bit tighter. The CrossFit definition of an athlete is "a person who is trained or skilled in strength, power, balance and agility, flexibility, and endurance." CrossFit holds "fitness," "health," and "athleticism" as strongly overlapping constructs. For most purposes, they can be seen as equivalents.

WHAT IF I DO NOT WANT TO BE AN ATHLETE; I JUST WANT TO BE HEALTHY?

You are in luck. We hear this often, but the truth is that fitness, wellness, and pathology (sickness) are measures of the same entity: your health. There are a multitude of measurable parameters that can be ordered from sick (pathological) to well (normal) to fit (better than normal). These include but are not limited to blood pressure, cholesterol, heart rate, body fat, muscle mass, flexibility, and strength. It seems as though all of the body functions that can go awry have states that are pathological, normal, and exceptional and that elite athletes typically show these parameters in the exceptional range. CrossFit's view is that fitness and health are the same thing (see "What Is Fitness? (Part 1)" article). It is also interesting to notice that the health professional maintains your health with drugs and surgery, each with potentially undesirable side effects, whereas the CrossFit trainer typically achieves a superior result always with "side benefit" versus side effect.

EXAMPLES OF CROSSFIT EXERCISES

Biking, running, swimming, and rowing in an endless variety of drills. The clean and jerk, snatch, squat, deadlift, push press, bench press, and power clean. Jumping, medicine-ball throws and catches, pull-ups, dips, push-ups, handstands, presses to handstands, pirouettes, kips, cartwheels, muscle-ups, sit-ups, scales, and holds. We make regular use of bikes, the track, rowing shells and ergometers, Olympic weight sets, rings, parallel bars, free exercise mats, horizontal bars, plyometrics boxes, medicine balls, and jump ropes.

There is not a strength and conditioning program anywhere that works with a greater diversity of tools, modalities, and drills.

WHAT IF I DO NOT HAVE TIME FOR ALL OF THIS?

It is a common sentiment to feel that because of the obligations of career and family that you do not have the time to become as fit as you might like. Here is the good news: World-class age group strength and conditioning is obtainable through an hour a day six days per week of training. It turns out that the intensity of training that optimizes physical conditioning is not sustainable past 45 minutes to an hour. Athletes who train for hours a day are developing skill or training for sports that include adaptations inconsistent with elite strength and conditioning. Past one hour, more is not better!

"FRINGE ATHLETES"

There is a near universal misconception that long-distance athletes are fitter than their short-distance counterparts. The triathlete, cyclist, and marathoner are often regarded as among the fittest athletes on Earth. Nothing could be further from the truth. The endurance athlete has trained long past any cardiovascular health benefit and has lost ground in strength, speed, and power; typically does nothing for coordination, agility, balance, and accuracy; and possesses little more than average flexibility. This is hardly the stuff of elite athleticism. The CrossFit athlete, remember, has trained and practiced for optimal physical competence in all 10 physical skills (cardiovascular/respiratory endurance, stamina, flexibility, strength, power, speed, coordination, agility, balance, and accuracy). The excessive aerobic volume of the endurance athletes' training costs them in speed, power, and strength to the point that their athletic competency has been compromised. No triathlete is in ideal shape to wrestle, box, pole-vault, sprint, play any ball sport, fight fires, or do police work. Each of these requires a fitness level far beyond the needs of the endurance athlete. None of this suggests that being a marathoner, triathlete or other endurance athlete is a bad thing; just do not believe that training as a long-distance athlete gives you the fitness that is prerequisite to many sports. CrossFit considers the sumo wrestler, triathlete, marathoner, and powerlifter to be "fringe athletes" in that their fitness demands are so specialized as to be inconsistent with the adaptations that give maximum competency at all physical challenges. Elite strength and conditioning is a compromise between each of the 10 physical adaptations. Endurance athletes do not balance that compromise.

AEROBICS AND ANAEROBICS

There are three main energy systems that fuel all human activity. Almost all changes that occur in the body due to exercise are related to the demands placed on these energy systems. Furthermore, the efficacy of any given fitness regimen may largely be tied to its ability to elicit an adequate stimulus for change within these three energy systems.

Energy is derived aerobically when oxygen is utilized to metabolize substrates derived from food and liberates energy. An activity is termed aerobic when the majority of energy needed is derived aerobically. These activities are usually greater than 90 seconds in duration and involve low to moderate power output or intensity. Examples of aerobic activity include running on the treadmill for 20 minutes, swimming a mile, and watching TV.

Energy is derived anaerobically when energy is liberated from substrates in the absence of oxygen. Activities are considered anaerobic when the majority of the energy needed is derived anaerobically. In fact, properly structured, anaerobic activity can be used to develop a very high level of aerobic fitness without the muscle wasting consistent with high-volume aerobic exercise! These activities are of less than two minutes in duration and involve moderate to high-power output or intensity. There are two such anaerobic systems, the phosphagen (or phosphocreatine) system and the lactic acid (or glycolytic) system. Examples of anaerobic activity include running a 100-meter sprint, squatting, and doing pull-ups.

Anaerobic and aerobic training support performance variables like strength, power, speed, and endurance. We also support the contention that total conditioning and optimal health necessitate training each of the physiological systems in a systematic fashion (see "What is Fitness? (Part 1)" article).

> "Traditionally, calisthenic movements are high-rep movements, but there are numerous body-weight exercises that only rarely can be performed for more than a rep or two. Find them. Explore them!"
>
> –COACH GLASSMAN

It warrants mention that in any activity all three energy systems are utilized though one may dominate. The interplay of these systems can be complex, yet a simple examination of the characteristics of aerobic versus anaerobic training can prove useful.

CrossFit's approach is to judiciously balance anaerobic and aerobic exercise in a manner that is consistent with the athlete's goals. Our exercise prescriptions adhere to proper specificity, progression, variation, and recovery to optimize adaptations.

THE OLYMPIC LIFTS, A.K.A., WEIGHTLIFTING

There are two Olympic lifts, the clean and jerk and the snatch. Mastery of these lifts develops the squat, deadlift, power clean, and split jerk while integrating them into a single movement of unequaled value in all of strength and conditioning. The Olympic lifters are without a doubt the world's strongest athletes.

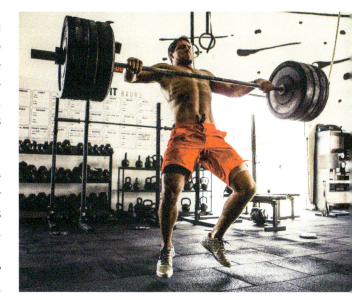

These lifts train athletes to effectively activate more muscle fibers more rapidly than through any other modality of training. The explosiveness that results from this training is of vital necessity to every sport.

Practicing the Olympic lifts teaches one to apply force to muscle groups in proper sequence; i.e., from the center of the body to its extremities (core to extremity). Learning this vital technical lesson benefits all athletes who need to impart force to another person or object, as is commonly required in nearly all sports.

In addition to learning to impart explosive forces, the clean and jerk and snatch condition the body to receive such forces from another moving body both safely and effectively.

Numerous studies have demonstrated the Olympic lifts' unique capacity to develop strength, muscle, power, speed, coordination, vertical leap, muscular endurance, bone strength, and the physical capacity to withstand stress. It is also worth mentioning that the Olympic lifts are the only lifts shown to increase maximum oxygen uptake, the most important marker for cardiovascular fitness.

Sadly, the Olympic lifts are seldom seen in the commercial fitness community because of their inherently complex and technical nature. CrossFit makes them available to anyone with the patience and persistence to learn.

GYMNASTICS

The extraordinary value of gymnastics as a training modality lies in its reliance on the body's own weight as the sole source of resistance. This places a unique premium on the improvement of strength-to-weight ratio. Unlike other strength training modalities, gymnastics and calisthenics allow for increases in strength only while increasing strength-to-weight ratio!

Gymnastics develops pull-ups, squats, lunges, jumping, push-ups, and numerous presses to handstand, scales, and holds. These skills are unrivaled in their benefit to the physique, as evident in any competitive gymnast.

As important as the capacity of this modality is for strength development, it is without a doubt the ultimate approach to improving coordination, balance, agility, accuracy, and flexibility. Through the use of numerous presses, handstands, scales, and other floor work, the gymnast's training greatly enhances kinesthetic sense.

The variety of movements available for inclusion in this modality probably exceeds the number of exercises known to all non-gymnastic sport! The rich variety here contributes substantially to CrossFit's ability to inspire great athletic confidence and prowess.

For a combination of strength, flexibility, well-developed physique, coordination, balance, accuracy, and agility, the gymnast has no equal in the sports world. The inclusion of this training modality is absurdly absent from nearly all training programs.

ROUTINES

There is no ideal routine! In fact, the chief value of any routine lies in abandoning it for another. The CrossFit ideal is to train for any contingency. The obvious implication is that this is possible only if there is a tremendously varied quality to the breadth of stimulus. It is in this sense that CrossFit is a core strength and conditioning program. Anything else is sport-specific training, not core strength and conditioning.

Any routine, no matter how complete, contains within its omissions the parameters for which there will be no adaptation. The breadth of adaptation will exactly match the breadth of the stimulus. For this reason, CrossFit embraces short-, middle-, and long-distance metabolic conditioning, and low, moderate, and heavy load assignment. We encourage creative and continuously varied compositions that tax physiological functions against every realistically conceivable combination of stressors. This is the stuff of surviving fights and fires. Developing a fitness that is varied yet complete defines the very art of strength and conditioning coaching.

This is not a comforting message in an age when scientific certainty and specialization confer authority and expertise. Yet, the reality of performance enhancement cares not one wit for trend or authority. CrossFit's success in elevating the performance of world-class athletes lies clearly in demanding of our athletes total and complete physical competence. No routine takes us there.

NEUROENDOCRINE ADAPTATION

"Neuroendocrine adaptation" is a change in the body that affects you either neurologically or hormonally. Most important adaptations to exercise are in part or completely a result of a hormonal or neurological shift. Research has shown which exercise protocols maximize neuroendocrine responses. Earlier we faulted isolation movements as being ineffectual. Now we can tell you that one of the critical elements missing from these movements is that they invoke essentially no neuroendocrine response.

Among the hormonal responses vital to athletic development are substantial increases in testosterone, insulin-like growth factor, and human growth hormone. Exercising with protocols known to elevate these hormones eerily mimics the hormonal changes sought in exogenous hormonal therapy (steroid use) with none of the deleterious effect. Exercise regimens that induce a high neuroendocrine response produce champions! Increased muscle mass and bone density are just two of many adaptive responses to exercises capable of producing a significant neuroendocrine response.

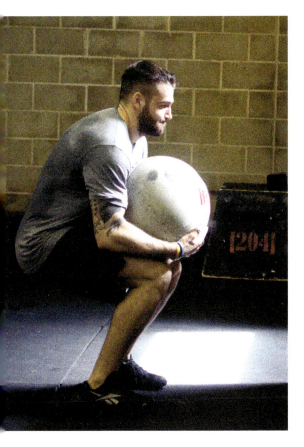

It is impossible to overstate the importance of the neuroendocrine response to exercise protocols. Heavy load weight training, short rest between sets, high heart rates, high-intensity training, and short rest intervals, though not entirely distinct components, are all associated with a high neuroendocrine response.

POWER

Power is defined as the "time rate of doing work." It has often been said that in sport speed is king. At CrossFit "power" is the undisputed king of performance. Power is, in simplest terms, "hard and fast." Jumping, punching, throwing, and sprinting are all measures of power. Increasing your ability to produce power is necessary and nearly sufficient to elite athleticism. Additionally, power is the definition of intensity, which in turn has been linked to nearly every positive aspect of fitness. Increases in strength, performance,

> "The CrossFit concept can be viewed as 'functional atomism' in that we strive to reduce human performance to a limited number of movements that are simple, irreducible, indivisible functions. Teaching an athlete to run, jump, throw, punch, squat, lunge, push, pull, and climb powerfully, with mechanical efficiency and soundness across a broad range of time-intensity protocols with rapid recovery establishes a foundation that will give unprecedented advantage in learning new sports, mastering existent skills, and surviving unforeseeable challenges."
>
> –COACH GLASSMAN

muscle mass, and bone density all arise in proportion to the intensity of exercise. And again, intensity is defined as power. Power development is an ever-present aspect of the CrossFit.com Workout of the Day (WOD).

CROSS TRAINING

Cross training is typically defined as participating in multiple sports. At CrossFit, we take a much broader view of the term. We view cross training as exceeding the normal parameters of the regular demands of your sport or training. CrossFit recognizes functional, metabolic, and modal cross training. That is,

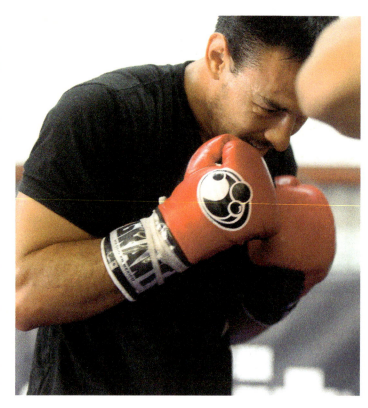

we regularly train past the normal motions, metabolic pathways, and modes or sports common to the athlete's sport or exercise regimen. We are unique and again distinctive to the extent that we adhere to and program within this context.

If you remember CrossFit's objective of providing a broad-based fitness that provides maximal competency in all adaptive capacities, then cross training, or training outside of the athlete's normal or regular demands, is a given. Long ago, we noticed that athletes are weakest at the margins of their exposure for almost every measurable parameter. For instance, if you only cycle between 5 and 7 miles at each training effort you will test weak at less than 5 and greater than 7 miles. This is true for range of motion, load, rest, intensity, power, etc. CrossFit workouts are engineered to expand the margins of exposure as broad as function and capacity will allow.

FUNCTIONAL MOVEMENTS

There are movements that mimic motor recruitment patterns that are found in everyday life. Others are somewhat unique to the gym. Squatting is standing from a seated position; deadlifting is picking any object off the ground. They are both functional movements. Leg extension and leg curl both have no equivalent in nature and are in turn non-functional movements. The bulk of isolation movements are non-functional movements. By contrast the compound or multi-joint movements are functional. Natural movement typically involves the movement of multiple joints for every activity.

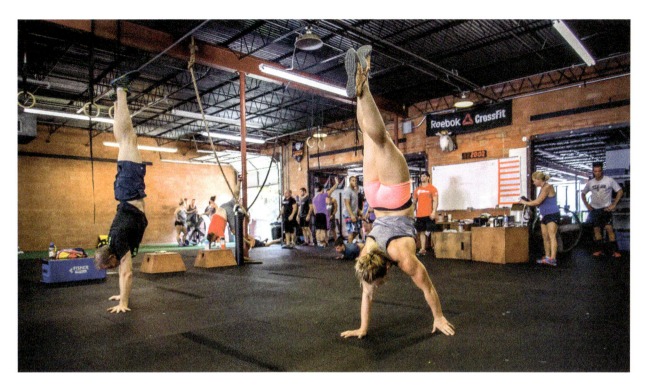

Functional movements are mechanically sound and therefore safe, and they also elicit a high neuroendocrine response.

CrossFit has managed a stable of elite athletes and dramatically enhanced their performance exclusively with functional movements. The superiority of training with functional movements is clearly apparent with any athlete within weeks of their incorporation.

The soundness and efficacy of functional movements are so profound that exercising without them is by comparison a colossal waste of time.

DIET

The CrossFit dietary prescription is as follows:
- Protein should be lean and varied and account for about 30 percent of your total caloric load.
- Carbohydrates should be predominantly low-glycemic and account for about 40 percent of your total caloric load.
- Fat should be from whole food sources and account for about 30 percent of your total caloric load.

Total calories should be based on protein needs, which should be set at between 0.7 and 1.0 grams of protein per pound of lean body mass (depending on your activity level). The 0.7 figure is for moderate daily workout loads, and the 1.0 figure is for the hardcore athlete.

WHAT SHOULD I EAT?

In plain language, base your diet on garden vegetables (especially greens), meats, nuts and seeds, some fruit, little starch, and no sugar. That is about as simple as we can get. Many have observed that keeping your grocery cart to the perimeter of the grocery store while avoiding the aisles is a great way to protect your health. Food is perishable. The stuff with long shelf life is all suspect. If you follow these simple guidelines, you will benefit from nearly all that can be achieved through nutrition.

THE CAVEMAN OR PALEOLITHIC MODEL FOR NUTRITION

Modern diets are ill suited for our genetic composition. Evolution has not kept pace with advances in agriculture and food processing, resulting in a plague of health problems for modern man. Coronary heart disease, diabetes, cancer, osteoporosis, obesity, and psychological dysfunction have all been scientifically linked to a diet too high in refined or processed carbohydrate. The caveman model is perfectly consistent with CrossFit's prescription.

WHAT FOODS SHOULD I AVOID?

Excessive consumption of high-glycemic carbohydrates is the primary culprit in nutritionally caused health problems. High-glycemic carbohydrates are those that raise blood sugar too rapidly. They include rice, bread, candy, potato, sweets, sodas, and most processed carbohydrates. Processing can include bleaching, baking, grinding, and refining. Processing of carbohydrates greatly increases their glycemic index, a measure of their propensity to elevate blood sugar.

WHAT IS THE PROBLEM WITH HIGH-GLYCEMIC CARBOHYDRATES?

The problem with high-glycemic carbohydrates is that in excess they give an inordinate insulin response. Insulin is an essential hormone for life, yet acute, chronic elevation of insulin leads to hyperinsulinism, which has been positively linked to obesity, elevated cholesterol levels, blood pressure, mood dysfunction, and a Pandora's box of disease and disability. Research "hyperinsulinism." CrossFit's prescription is a low-glycemic diet (and relatively lower in total carbohydrate quantity) and consequently severely blunts the insulin response, yet still provides ample nutrition for rigorous activity. ▪

WHAT IS FITNESS? (PART 1)

Originally published in October 2002. This article explains the supporting models and concepts for defining fitness, which was formally codified years after this publication. "What Is Fitness? (Part 2)," which follows, contains the definitions of fitness and health.

WHAT IS FITNESS AND WHO IS FIT?

In 1997, Outside Magazine crowned triathlete Mark Allen "the fittest man on Earth." Let us just assume for a moment that this famous six-time winner of the Ironman Triathlon is the fittest of the fit, then what title do we bestow on the decathlete Simon Poelman, who also possesses incredible endurance and stamina, yet crushes Mr. Allen in any comparison that includes strength, power, speed, and coordination?

Perhaps the definition of fitness does not include strength, speed, power, and co-ordination, though that seems rather odd. Merriam Webster's Collegiate Dictionary defines "fitness" and being "fit" as the ability to transmit genes and being healthy. No help there. Searching the internet for a workable, reasonable definition of fitness yields disappointingly little. Worse yet, the National Strength and Conditioning Association (NSCA), the most respected publisher in exercise physiology, in its highly authoritative "Essentials of Strength Training and Conditioning," does not even attempt a definition.

CROSSFIT'S FITNESS

For CrossFit, the specter of championing a fitness program without clearly defining what it is that the program delivers combines elements of fraud and farce. The vacuum of guiding authority has therefore necessitated that CrossFit provides its own definition of fitness. That is what this article is about: our "fitness."

Our pondering, studying, debating about, and finally defining fitness have played a formative role in Cross-Fit's successes. The keys to understanding the methods and achievements of CrossFit are perfectly embedded in our view of fitness and basic exercise science.

It will come as no surprise to most of you that our view of fitness is a contrarian view. The general public both in opinion and in media holds endurance athletes as exemplars of fitness. We do not. Our incredulity on learning of Outside's awarding a triathlete the title of "fittest man on Earth" becomes apparent in light of CrossFit's models for assessing and defining fitness.

Eat meat and vegetables, nuts and seeds, some fruit, little starch, and no sugar. Keep intake to levels that will support exercise but not body fat.

Practice and train major lifts: Deadlift, clean, squat, presses, C&J (clean and jerk), and snatch. Similarly, master the basics of gymnastics: pull-ups, dips, rope climbs, push-ups, sit-ups, presses to handstands, pirouettes, flips, splits, and holds. Bike, run, swim, row, etc. hard and fast.

Five or six days per week mix these elements in as many combinations and patterns as creativity will allow. Routine is the enemy. Keep workouts short and intense.

Regularly learn and play new sports.

Figure 1. World-Class Fitness in 100 Words.

CrossFit makes use of four different models for evaluating and guiding fitness. Collectively, these four models provide the basis for CrossFit's definition of fitness. The first is based on the 10 general physical skills widely recognized by exercise physiologists; the second model is based on the performance of athletic tasks; the third is based on the energy systems that drive all human action; the fourth uses health markers as a measure of fitness.

Each model is critical to CrossFit and each has distinct utility in evaluating an athlete's overall fitness or a strength and conditioning regimen's efficacy. Before explaining in detail how each of these four models works, it warrants mention that we are not attempting to demonstrate our program's legitimacy through scientific principles. We are but sharing the methods of a program whose legitimacy has been established through the testimony of athletes, soldiers, cops, and others whose lives or livelihoods depend on fitness.

If your goal is optimum physical competence, then all the general physical skills must be considered:

1. Cardiovascular/respiratory endurance–The ability of body systems to gather, process, and deliver oxygen.

2. Stamina–The ability of body systems to process, deliver, store, and utilize energy.

3. Strength–The ability of a muscular unit, or combination of muscular units, to apply force.

4. Flexibility–The ability to maximize the range of motion at a given joint.

5. Power–The ability of a muscular unit, or combination of muscular units, to apply maximum force in minimum time.

6. Speed–The ability to minimize the time cycle of a repeated movement.

7. Coordination–The ability to combine several distinct movement patterns into a singular distinct movement.

8. Agility–The ability to minimize transition time from one movement pattern to another.

9. Balance–The ability to control the placement of the body's center of gravity in relation to its support base.

10. Accuracy–The ability to control movement in a given direction or at a given intensity.

(Thanks to Jim Cawley and Bruce Evans of Dynamax)

Figure 2. Ten General Physical Skills.

CROSSFIT'S FIRST FITNESS MODEL: THE 10 GENERAL PHYSICAL SKILLS

There are 10 recognized general physical skills. They are cardiovascular/respiratory endurance, stamina, strength, flexibility, power, speed, coordination, agility, balance, and accuracy. (See Figure 2. Ten General Physical Skills for definitions.) You are as fit as you are competent in each of these 10 skills. A regimen develops fitness to the extent that it improves each of these 10 skills.

Importantly, improvements in endurance, stamina, strength, and flexibility come about through training. Training refers to activity that improves performance through a measurable organic change in the body. By contrast improvements in coordination, agility, balance, and accuracy come about through practice. Practice refers to activity that improves performance through changes in the nervous system. Power and speed are adaptations of both training and practice.

TABLE 1. SUMMARY OF THE THREE METABOLIC PATHWAYS			
	Phosphagen	**Glycolytic**	**Oxidative**
Time Domain	Short, ~10 seconds	Medium, ~120 seconds	Long, >120 seconds
Anaerobic vs. Aerobic	Anaerobic	Anaerobic	Aerobic
Relative Power Output	Maximum-intensity efforts (~100 percent)	Medium-high-intensity efforts (70 percent)	Low-intensity efforts (40 percent)
Other Names	Phosphocreatine	Lactate	Aerobic
Location	Cytosol of muscle cells (i.e., sarcoplasm)	Cytosol of all cells	Mitochondria of cells
Muscle Fiber Type (General)	Type IIb	Type IIa	Type I
Substrate	Phosphocreatine molecules in muscles	Glucose from bloodstream, muscle (glycogen), or glycerol (derived from fat)	Pyruvate (from glycolysis), or acetate (derived from fat or protein)
ATP Mechanism	Phosphate molecule from phosphocreatine joins ADP to form ATP	Glucose oxidized to pyruvate produces 2 ATP	Pyruvate oxidized to produce 34 ATP (fat, protein yield less)
Example Activities	100-meter dash 1-repetition-maximum deadlift	400-meter sprint Elite-level Fran	Anything >120 seconds of sustained effort

Our emphasis on skill development is integral to our charter of optimizing work capacity."

–COACH GLASSMAN

CROSSFIT'S SECOND FITNESS MODEL: THE HOPPER

The essence of this model is the view that fitness is about performing well at any and every task imaginable. Picture a hopper loaded with an infinite number of physical challenges, where no selective mechanism is operative, and being asked to perform feats randomly drawn from the hopper. This model suggests that your fitness can be measured by your capacity to perform well at these tasks in relation to other individuals.

The implication here is that fitness requires an ability to perform well at all tasks, even unfamiliar tasks and tasks combined in infinitely varying combinations. In practice this encourages the athlete to disinvest in any set notions of sets, rest periods, reps, exercises, order of exercises, routines, periodization, etc. Nature frequently

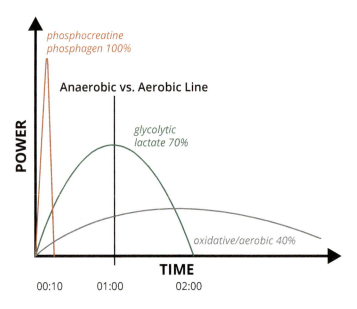

Figure 3. Potential Power Output Versus Duration for the Three Metabolic Energy Pathways.

provides largely unforeseeable challenges; train for that by striving to keep the training stimulus broad and constantly varied.

CROSSFIT'S THIRD FITNESS MODEL: THE METABOLIC PATHWAYS
There are three metabolic pathways that provide the energy for all human action. These "metabolic engines" are known as the phosphagen (or phosphocreatine) pathway, the glycolytic (or lactate) pathway, and the oxidative (or aerobic) pathway (Table 1, Figure 3). The first, the phosphagen, dominates the highest-powered activities, those that last less than about 10 seconds. The second pathway, the glycolytic, dominates moderate-powered activities, those that last up to several minutes. The third pathway, the oxidative, dominates low-powered activities, those that last in excess of several minutes.

Total fitness, the fitness that CrossFit promotes and develops, requires competency and training in each of these three pathways or engines. Balancing the effects of these three pathways largely determines the how and why of the metabolic conditioning or "cardio" that we do at CrossFit.

Favoring one or two to the exclusion of the others and not recognizing the impact of excessive training in the oxidative pathway are arguably the two most common faults in fitness training. More on that later.

CROSSFIT'S FOURTH FITNESS MODEL: SICKNESS-WELLNESS-FITNESS CONTINUUM
There is another aspect to CrossFit's fitness that is of great interest and immense value to us. We have observed that nearly every measurable value of health can be

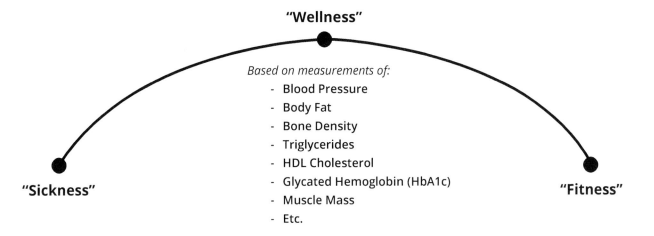

Figure 4. The Sickness-Wellness-Fitness Continuum.

placed on a continuum that ranges from sickness to wellness to fitness (Figure 4). Though tougher to measure, we would even add mental health to this observation. Depression is clearly mitigated by proper diet and exercise.

For example, a blood pressure of 160/95 is pathological, 120/70 is normal or healthy, and 105/55 is consistent with an athlete's blood pressure; a body fat of 40 percent is pathological, 20 percent is normal or healthy, and 10 percent is fit. We observe a similar ordering for bone density, triglycerides, muscle mass, flexibility, high-density lipoprotein (HDL) or "good cholesterol," resting heart rate, and dozens of other common measures of health (Table 2). Many authorities (e.g., Mel Siff, the NSCA) make a clear distinction between health and fitness. Frequently they cite studies that suggest that the fit may not be health protected. A close look at the supporting evidence invariably reveals the studied group is endurance athletes and, we suspect, endurance athletes on a dangerous fad diet (high carbohydrate, low fat, low protein).

Done right, fitness provides a great margin of protection against the ravages of time and disease. Where you find otherwise, examine the fitness protocol, especially diet. Fitness is and should be "super-wellness." Sickness, wellness, and fitness are measures of the same entity. A fitness regimen that does not support health is not CrossFit.

COMMON GROUND
The motivation for the four models is simply to ensure the broadest and most general fitness possible. Our first model evaluates our efforts against a full range of general physical adaptations; in the second the focus is on breadth and depth of performance; with the third the measure is time, power and consequently energy systems; and the fourth is on health markers. It should be fairly clear that the fitness that CrossFit advocates and develops is deliberately broad, general, and inclusive. Our specialty is not specializing. Combat, survival, many sports, and life reward this kind of fitness and, on average, punish the specialist.

TABLE 2. REPRESENTATIVE SICKNESS-WELLNESS-FITNESS VALUES FOR SELECTED PARAMETERS			
Parameter	Sickness	Wellness	Fitness
Body Fat (percent)	>25 (male) >32 (female)	~18 (male) ~20 (female)	~6 (male) ~12 (female)
Blood Pressure (mm/Hg)	>140/90	120/80	105/60
Resting Heart Rate (bpm)	>100	70	50
Triglycerides (mg/dL)	>200	<150	<100
Low-density Lipoprotein (mg/dL)	>160	120	<100
High-density Lipoprotein (mg/dL)	<40	40-59	>60
C-Reactive Protein (high-sensitivity test, mg/L)	>3	1-3	<1

IMPLEMENTATION

Our fitness, being "CrossFit," comes through molding men and women who are equal parts gymnast, Olympic weightlifter, and multi-modal sprinter or "sprintathlete." Develop the capacity of a novice 800-meter track athlete, gymnast, and weightlifter, and you will be fitter than any world-class runner, gymnast, or weightlifter. Let us look at how CrossFit incorporates metabolic conditioning ("cardio"), gymnastics, and weightlifting to forge the world's fittest men and women.

METABOLIC CONDITIONING, OR "CARDIO"

Biking, running, swimming, rowing, speed skating, and cross-country skiing are collectively known as "metabolic conditioning." In the common vernacular they are referred to as "cardio." CrossFit's third fitness model, the one that deals with metabolic pathways, contains the seeds of the CrossFit "cardio" prescription. To understand the CrossFit approach to "cardio" we need first to briefly cover the nature and interaction of the three major pathways.

Of the three metabolic pathways the first two, the phosphagen and the glycolytic, are "anaerobic" and the third, the oxidative, is "aerobic." We need not belabor the biochemical significance of aerobic and anaerobic systems; suffice it to say that understanding the nature and interaction of anaerobic exercise and aerobic exercise is vital to understanding conditioning. Just remember that efforts at moderate to high power and lasting less than several minutes are predominantly anaerobic and efforts at low power and lasting in excess of several minutes are predominantly aerobic. As an example, the sprints at 100, 200, 400, and 800 meters are largely anaerobic and events like 1,500 meters, the mile, 2,000 meters, and 3,000 meters are largely aerobic.

Aerobic training benefits cardiovascular function and decreases body fat—all good. Aerobic conditioning allows us to engage in low-power extended efforts efficiently (cardio/respiratory endurance and stamina). This is critical to many sports. Athletes engaged in sports or training where a preponderance of the training load is spent in aerobic efforts witness decreases in muscle mass, strength, speed, and power. It is not uncommon to find marathoners with a vertical leap of only several inches! Furthermore, aerobic activity has a pronounced tendency to decrease anaerobic capacity. This does not bode well for most athletes or those interested in elite fitness.

Anaerobic activity also benefits cardiovascular function and decreases body fat! In fact, anaerobic exercise is superior to aerobic exercise for fat loss! Anaerobic activity is, however, unique in its capacity to dramatically improve power, speed, strength, and muscle mass. Anaerobic conditioning allows us to exert tremendous forces over brief time intervals. One aspect of anaerobic conditioning that bears great consideration is that anaerobic conditioning will not adversely affect aerobic capacity. In fact, properly structured, anaerobic activity can be used to develop a very high level of aerobic fitness without the muscle wasting consistent with high volumes of aerobic exercise! The method by which we use anaerobic efforts to develop aerobic conditioning is "interval training."

Basketball, football, gymnastics, boxing, track events under one mile, soccer, swimming events under 400 meters, volleyball, wrestling, and weightlifting are all sports that require the vast majority of training time to be spent in anaerobic activity. Long-distance and ultra- endurance running, cross-country skiing, and 1,500+ meter swimming are all sports that require aerobic training at levels that produce results unacceptable to other athletes or the individual concerned with total conditioning and optimal health.

We strongly recommend that you attend a track meet of nationally or internationally competitive athletes. Pay close attention to the physiques of the athletes competing at 100, 200, 400, and 800 meters and the milers. The difference you are sure to notice is a direct result of training at those distances.

INTERVAL TRAINING

The key to developing the cardiovascular system without an unacceptable loss of strength, speed, and power is interval training. Interval training mixes bouts of work and rest in timed intervals. Table 3 gives guidelines for interval training. We can control the dominant metabolic pathway conditioned by varying the duration of the work and rest interval and number of interval repetitions. Note that the phosphagen pathway is the dominant pathway in intervals of 10–30 seconds of work followed by rest of 30–90 seconds (work:recovery 1:3) repeated 25–30 times. The glycolytic pathway is the dominant pathway in intervals of 30–120 seconds of work followed by rest of 60–240 seconds (work:recovery 1:2) repeated 10–20

Blur the distinction between strength training and metabolic conditioning for the simple reason that nature's challenges are typically blind to the distinction."

–COACH GLASSMAN

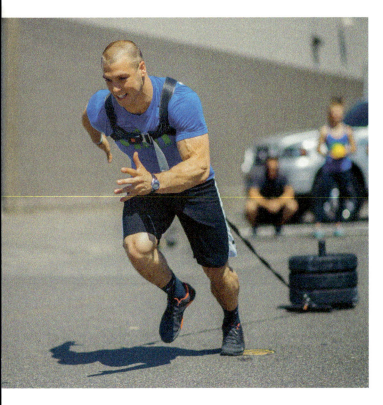

times. And finally, the oxidative pathway is the dominant pathway in intervals of 120–300 seconds of work followed by rest of 120–300 seconds (work:recovery 1:1) repeated 3–5 times. The bulk of metabolic training should be interval training.

Interval training need not be so structured or formal. One example would be to sprint between one set of telephone poles and jog between the next set, alternating in this manner for the duration of a run.

One example of an interval that CrossFit makes regular use of is the Tabata interval, which is 20 seconds of work followed by 10 seconds of rest repeated eight times. Dr. Izumi Tabata published research that demonstrated that this interval protocol produced remarkable increases in both anaerobic and aerobic capacity.

It is highly desirable to regularly experiment with interval patterns of varying combinations of rest, work, and repetitions.

Some of the best resources on interval training come from Dr. Stephen Seiler. His articles on interval training and the time course of training adaptations contain the seeds of CrossFit's heavy reliance on interval training. The article on the time course of training adaptations explains that there are three waves of adaptation to endurance training. The first wave is increased maximal oxygen consumption. The second is increased lactate threshold. The third is increased efficiency. In the CrossFit concept, we are interested in maximizing first-wave adaptations and procuring the second systemically through multiple modalities, including weight training, and avoiding completely third-wave adaptations. Second- and third-wave adaptations are highly specific to the activity in which they are developed and can be detrimental with too much focus to the broad fitness that we advocate and develop. A clear understanding of this material has prompted us to advocate regular high-intensity training in as many training modalities as possible through largely anaerobic efforts and intervals while deliberately and specifically avoiding the efficiency that accompanies mastery of a single modality. It is at first ironic that our interpretation of Dr. Seiler's work was not his intention, but when our quest of optimal physical competence is viewed in light of Dr. Seiler's more specific aim of maximizing endurance performance, our interpretation is powerful.

TABLE 3. REPRESENTATIVE GUIDELINES FOR INTERVAL TRAINING			
Primary Energy System	**Phosphagen**	**Glycolytic**	**Oxidative**
Duration of work (in seconds)	10–30	30–120	120–300
Duration of recovery (in seconds)	30–90	60–240	120–300
Work:recovery ratio	1:3	1:2	1:1
Total interval repetitions	25–30	10–20	3–5

Dr. Seiler's work, incidentally, makes clear the fallacy of assuming that endurance work is of greater benefit to the cardiovascular system than higher intensity interval work. This is very important: with interval training we get all of the cardiovascular benefit of endurance work without the attendant loss of strength, speed, and power.

GYMNASTICS

Our use of the term "gymnastics" not only includes the traditional competitive sport that we have seen on TV but all activities like climbing, yoga, calisthenics, and dance, where the aim is body control. It is within this realm of activities that we can develop extraordinary strength (especially upper body and trunk), flexibility, coordination, balance, agility, and accuracy. In fact, the traditional gymnast has no peer in terms of development of these skills.

CrossFit uses short parallel bars, mats, still rings, pull-up and dip bars, and a climbing rope to implement our gymnastics training.

The starting place for gymnastic competency lies with the well-known calisthenic movements: pull-ups, push-ups, dips, and rope climbs. These movements need to form the core of your upper-body strength work. Set goals for achieving benchmarks like 20, 25, and 30 pull-ups; 50, 75, and 100 push-ups; 20, 30, 40, and 50 dips; 1, 2, 3, 4, and 5 consecutive trips up the rope without any use of the feet or legs.

At 15 pull-ups and dips each, it is time to start working regularly on a "muscle-up." The muscle-up is moving from a hanging position below the rings to a supported position, arms extended, above the rings. It is a combination movement containing both a pull-up and a dip. Far from a contrivance, the muscle-up is hugely functional. With a muscle-up, you will be able to surmount any object on which you can get a finger hold—if you can touch it, you can get up on it. The value here for survival, police, firefighter, and military use is impossible to overstate. Pull-ups and dips are the key to developing the muscle-up.

While developing your upper-body strength with the pull-ups, push-ups, dips, and rope climbs, a large measure of balance and accuracy can be developed through mastering the handstand. Start with a headstand against the wall if you need to. Once reasonably comfortable with the inverted position of the headstand, you can practice kicking up to the handstand again against a wall. Later take the handstand to the short parallel bars or parallettes without the benefit of the wall. After you can hold a handstand for several minutes without benefit of the wall or a spotter it is time to develop a pirouette. A pirouette is lifting one arm and turning on the supporting arm 90 degrees to regain the handstand, then repeating this with alternate arms until you have turned 180 degrees. This skill needs to be practiced until it can be done with little chance of falling from the handstand. Work in intervals of 90 degrees as benchmarks of your growth—90, 180, 270, 360, 450, 540, 630, and finally 720 degrees.

> **"**
>
> Much of the rudiments of gymnastics come only with great effort and frustration—that is acceptable."
>
> –COACH GLASSMAN

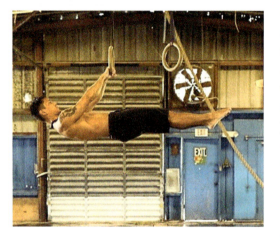

Walking on the hands is another fantastic tool for developing both the handstand and balance and accuracy. A football field or sidewalk is an excellent place to practice and measure your progress. You want to be able to walk 100 yards in the handstand without falling.

Competency in the handstand readies the athlete for handstand presses. There is a family of presses that range from relatively easy ones that any beginning gymnast can perform to ones so difficult that only the best gymnasts competing at national levels can perform. Their hierarchy of difficulty is bent arm/bent body (hip)/bent leg; straight arm/bent body/bent leg; straight arm/bent body/straight leg; and bent arm/straight body/straight leg; and finally the monster: straight arm/straight body/straight leg. It is not unusual to take 10 years to get these five presses!

The trunk flexion work in gymnastics is beyond anything you will see anywhere else. Even the beginning gymnastics trunk movements cripple bodybuilders, weightlifters, and martial artists. The basic sit-up and "L" hold are the staples. The L-hold is nothing more than holding your trunk straight while supported by locked arms with hands on a bench, the floor or parallel bars; the hips are kept at 90 degrees with legs straight out in front of you. You want to work towards a three-minute hold in benchmark increments of 30 seconds—30, 60, 90, 120, 150, and 180 seconds. When you can hold an "L" for three minutes, all your old ab work will be silly easy.

We recommend Bob Anderson's "Stretching." This is a simple, no nonsense approach to flexibility. The science of stretching is weakly developed, and many athletes, like gymnasts who demonstrate great flexibility, receive no formal instruction. Just do it. Generally, you want to stretch in a warm-up to establish safe, effective range of motion for the ensuing activity and stretch during cool down to improve flexibility.

There is a lot of material to work with here. We highly recommend an adult gymnastics program if there is one in your area. Our friends at Drills and Skills have enough material to keep you busy for years. This is among our favorite fitness sites.

Every workout should contain regular gymnastic/calisthenic movements that you have mastered and other elements under development. Much of the rudiments of gymnastics come only with great effort and frustration—that is acceptable. The return is unprecedented and the most frustrating elements are most beneficial—long before you have developed even a modicum of competency.

WEIGHTLIFTING

"Weightlifting" as opposed to "weight lifting" or "weight training," refers to the Olympic sport, which includes the "clean and jerk" and the "snatch." Weightlifting, as it is often referred to, develops strength (especially in the hips), speed, and power like no other training modality. It is little known that successful weightlifting requires substantial flexibility. Olympic weightlifters are as flexible as any athletes.

The benefits of weightlifting do not end with strength, speed, power, and flexibility. The clean and jerk and the snatch both develop coordination, agility, accuracy, and balance and to no small degree. Both of these lifts are as nuanced and challenging as any movement in all of sport. Moderate competency in the Olympic lifts confers added prowess to any sport.

The Olympic lifts are based on the deadlift, clean, squat, and jerk. These movements are the starting point for any serious weight-training program. In fact they should serve as the core of your resistance training throughout your life.

Why the deadlift, clean, squat, and jerk? Because these movements elicit a profound neuroendocrine response. That is, they alter you hormonally and neurologically. The changes that occur through these movements are essential to athletic development. Most of the

If strength at high heart rates is fundamental to your sport then you'd best perform your resistance training at high heart rate."

–COACH GLASSMAN

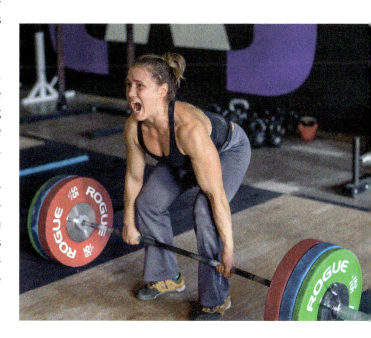

development that occurs as a result of exercise is systemic and a direct result of hormonal and neurological changes.

Curls, lateral raises, leg extensions, leg curls, flyes, and other bodybuilding movements have no place in a serious strength and conditioning program primarily because they have a blunted neuroendocrine response. A distinctive feature of these relatively worthless movements is that they have no functional analog in everyday life and they work only one joint at a time. Compare this to the deadlift, clean, squat, and jerk, which are functional and multi-joint movements.

Start your weightlifting career with the deadlift, clean, squat, and jerk, then introduce the clean and jerk and snatch. Much of the best weight-training material on the internet is found on powerlifting sites. Powerlifting is the sport of three lifts: the bench press, squat, and deadlift. Powerlifting is a superb start to a lifting program followed later by the more dynamic clean and the jerk and finally the clean and jerk and the snatch.

The movements that we are recommending are very demanding and very athletic. As a result they have kept athletes interested and intrigued where the typical fare offered in most gyms (bodybuilding movements) typically bores athletes to distraction. Weightlifting is sport; weight training is not.

THROWING
Our program includes not only weightlifting and powerlifting but also throwing work with medicine balls. The medicine-ball work we favor provides both physical training and general movement practice. We are huge fans of the Dynamax medicine ball and associated throwing exercises. The medicine-ball drills add another potent stimulus for strength, power, speed, coordination, agility, balance, and accuracy.

There is a medicine-ball game known as Hoover-Ball. It is played with an 8-foot volleyball net and scored like tennis. This game burns three times more calories than tennis and is great fun. The history and rules of Hoover-Ball are available from the internet.

NUTRITION
Nutrition plays a critical role in your fitness. Proper nutrition can amplify or diminish the effect of your training efforts. Effective nutrition is moderate in protein, carbohydrate, and fat. Forget about the fad high-carbohydrate, low-fat, and low-protein diet. Balanced macronutrient and healthy nutrition looks more like 40 percent carbohydrate, 30 percent protein, and 30 percent fat. Dr. Barry Sears' Zone Diet still offers the greatest precision, efficacy, and health benefit of any clearly defined protocol. The Zone Diet does an adequate job of jointly managing issues of blood glucose control, proper macronutrient proportion, and caloric restriction whether your concern is athletic performance, disease prevention and longevity,

> There is no single sport or activity that trains for perfect fitness. True fitness requires a compromise in adaptation broader than the demands of most every sport."
>
> –COACH GLASSMAN

or body composition. We recommend that everyone read Dr. Sears' book "Enter the Zone" (see also "Zone Meal Plans" article).

SPORT

Sport plays a wonderful role in fitness. Sport is the application of fitness in a fantastic atmosphere of competition and mastery. Training efforts typically include relatively predictable repetitive movements and provide limited opportunity for the essential combination of our 10 general physical skills. It is, after all, the combined expression, or application, of the 10 general skills that is our motivation for their development in the first place. Sports and games like soccer, martial arts, baseball, and basketball, in contrast to our training workouts, have more varied and less predictable movements. But, where sports develop and require all 10 general skills simultaneously, they do so slowly compared to our strength and conditioning regimen. Sport is better, in our view, at expression and testing of skills than it is at developing these same skills. Both expression and development are crucial to our fitness. Sport, in many respects, more closely mimics the demands of nature than does our training. We encourage and expect our athletes to engage in regular sports efforts in addition to all of their strength and conditioning work.

A THEORETICAL HIERARCHY OF DEVELOPMENT

A theoretical hierarchy exists for the development of an athlete (Figure 5). It starts with nutrition and moves to metabolic conditioning, gymnastics, weightlifting, and finally sport. This hierarchy largely reflects foundational dependence, skill, and to some degree, time ordering of development. The logical flow is from molecular foundations to cardiovascular sufficiency, body control, external object control, and ultimately mastery and application. This model has greatest utility in analyzing athletes' shortcomings or difficulties.

We do not deliberately order these components but nature will. If you have a deficiency at any level of "the pyramid" the components above will suffer.

INTEGRATION

Every regimen, every routine contains within its structure a blueprint for its deficiency. If you only work your weight training at low reps you will not develop the localized muscular endurance that you might have otherwise. If you work high reps exclusively you will not build the same strength or power that you would have at low reps. There are advantages and disadvantages to working out slowly or quickly, with high weights or low weights, completing "cardio" before or after, etc.

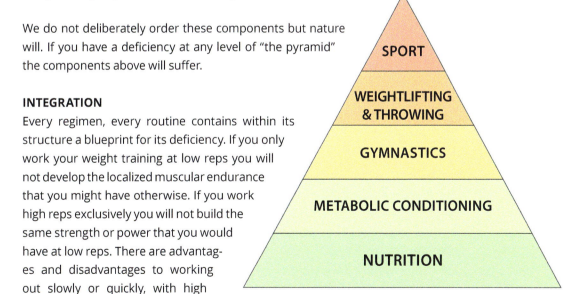

Figure 5. The Theoretical Hierarchy of the Development of an Athlete.

The needs of an Olympic athlete and our grandparents differ by degree not kind."

–COACH GLASSMAN

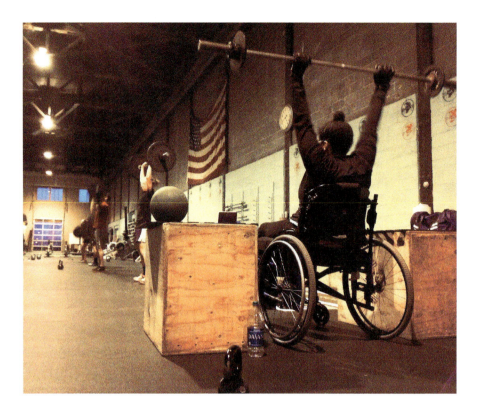

For the fitness that we are pursuing, every parameter within your control needs to be modulated to broaden the stimulus as much as possible. Your body will only respond to an unaccustomed stressor; routine is the enemy of progress and broad adaptation. Do not subscribe to high reps, or low reps, or long rests, or short rests but strive for variance.

So then, what are we to do? Work on becoming a better weightlifter, stronger-better gymnast, and faster rower, runner, swimmer, cyclist is the answer. There are an infinite number of workouts that will deliver the goods.

Generally, we have found that three days on and one day off allows for a maximum sustainability at maximum intensities. One of our favorite workout patterns is to warm up and then perform 3 to 5 sets of 3 to 5 reps of a fundamental lift at a moderately comfortable pace followed by a 10-minute circuit of gymnastics elements at a blistering pace and finally finish with 2 to 10 minutes of high-intensity metabolic conditioning. There is nothing sacred in this pattern. The magic is in the movements not the routine. Be creative.

Another favorite is to blend elements of gymnastics and weightlifting in couplets that combine to make a dramatic metabolic challenge. An example would be to perform 5 reps of a moderately heavy back squat followed immediately by a set of max-reps pull-ups repeated 3–5 times.

On other occasions we will take five or six elements balanced between weightlifting, metabolic conditioning, and gymnastics and combine them in a single circuit that we blow through three times without a break.

We can create routines like this forever. In fact, our CrossFit.com archives contain thousands of daily workouts consciously mixed and varied in this manner. Perusing them will give you an idea of how we mix and modulate our key elements.

We have not mentioned here our penchant for jumping, kettlebells, odd-object lifting, and obstacle-course work. The recurring theme of functionality and variety clearly suggest the need and validity for their inclusion though.

Finally, strive to blur distinctions between "cardio" and strength training. Nature has no regard for this distinction or any other, including our 10 physical adaptations. We will use weights and plyometrics training to elicit a metabolic response and sprinting to improve strength.

SCALABILITY AND APPLICABILITY

The question regularly arises as to the applicability of a regimen like CrossFit's to older and deconditioned or untrained populations. The needs of an Olympic athlete and our grandparents differ by degree not kind. One is looking for functional dominance, the other for functional competence. Competence and dominance manifest through identical physiological mechanisms.

We have used our same routines for elderly individuals with heart disease and cage fighters one month out from televised bouts. We scale load and intensity; we do not change programs.

We get requests from athletes from every sport looking for a strength and conditioning program for their sport. Firemen, soccer players, triathletes, boxers, and surfers all want programs that conform to the specificity of their needs. While we admit that there are surely needs specific to any sport, the bulk of sport-specific training has been ridiculously ineffective. The need for specificity is nearly completely met by regular practice and training within the sport, not in the strength and conditioning environment. Our terrorist hunters, skiers, mountain bikers and housewives have found their best fitness from the same regimen. ▪

WHAT IS FITNESS? (PART 2)

Adapted from Coach Glassman's Feb 21, 2009, L1 lecture.

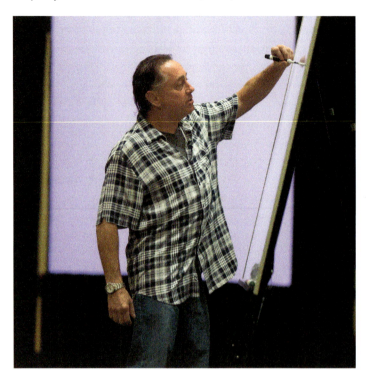

This concept started with me having what I call "a belief in fitness."

I was (and still am) of the view that there is a physical capacity that would lend itself generally well to any and all contingencies—to the likely, to the unlikely, to the known, to the unknown. This physical capacity is different than the fitness required for sport. One of the things that demarcates sport is how much we know about the event's physiological demands. Instead, we are chasing headlong this concept of fitness—as a broad, general and inclusive adaptive capacity—a fitness that would prepare you for the unknown and the unknowable.

And we went to the literature to look for such a definition and could not find anything. The information we did find seemed esoteric, irrelevant, or flawed—logically and/or scientifically. For example, to date the American College of Sports Medicine (ACSM) cannot give a scientific definition of fitness. They give a definition, but it contains nothing that can be measured. If it is not measurable, it is not a valid definition.

THE FIRST THREE MODELS

And so we started playing with a definition and came out with three operational models. They were clumsy, but they had utility: They guided us and kept us on this path towards this fitness.

The first model originated from Jim Cawley and Bruce Evans of Dynamax medicine balls. They produced a list of physiological adaptations that represented the gamut of potential physiological adaptations in an exercise program. You can improve cardiorespiratory endurance, stamina, strength, flexibility, power, speed, coordination, accuracy, agility and balance by exercising. They gave reasonable definitions to each of these 10 so that they seemed fairly distinct. Keep in mind, however, nature has no obligation to recognize these distinctions. They are completely manmade. This model is an abstraction to help us understand fitness better.

What we did with this was we said that a person was as fit as he or she was developed in breadth and depth in those 10 capacities. And to the extent that he or she was deficient in one capacity relative to any cohort, he or she was less fit. This is a balance: a compromise of physiological adaptation.

The second model is a statistical model based on training modality. A hopper, like those used to determine a lottery winner, is loaded with as many skills and drills from as many different sports and strength and conditioning regimens imaginable. It could be agility drills from track; one-rep-max bench press from football; Fran, Helen and Diane from CrossFit; Pilates, and yoga. Do not exclude anything: the more, the better. Then, line up everyone willing to participate, turn the handle, pull a task out at random, and put them to the test. Here is the contention: he or she who performs best at these randomly assigned physical tasks is the fittest.

It may very well be that the fittest man on Earth is in the 75th percentile for each event picked. In fact, being best at many things would tell me immediately that you are not as fit as you could be.

For instance, if you have a 4-minute mile time, thousands of people are much fitter than you. Part of the adaptation to get a 4-minute mile is that it coincides with the max bench press of about half body weight and a vertical leap of 3 to 4 inches. That is part and parcel of the adaptation. It is not a character flaw. There is no value judgment. Rather, you are not advancing your fitness. Instead, you are advancing a very narrow bandwidth of a specialized capacity.

Everyone probably knows what it is he or she does not want to see come out of the hopper. What I have learned about fitness, about sport training, about preparing yourself for the unknown and the unknowable is this: There is more traction, more advantage, more opportunity in pursuing headlong that event or skill that you do not want to see come out of the hopper than putting more time into the ones where you already excel. That thing you do not want to see come out of the hopper is a chink in your armor. It is a glaring deficiency in your general physical preparedness (GPP). And fixing it will give advantage where it does not always make sense maybe mechanically or metabolically.

Valid criticisms of a fitness program need to speak to measurable, observable, repeatable data. If an alternative to CrossFit is worthy of our consideration it ought to be presented in terms of distance, time, load, velocity, work and power related to movements, skills, and drills. Give me performance data. CrossFit can be scientifically and logically evaluated only on these terms."

–COACH GLASSMAN

We have countless examples of this from amateur and professional sports. At the heart of this is that we have learned some things about GPP that the world never knew before. There is more opportunity of advancing athletic performance via advancing GPP than there is in more sport-specific strength and conditioning training. For example, I am not sure why more pull-ups make for better skiers, but they do. We have some theories why that occurs, but we do not actually need to know the mechanism. We are focused on advancing performance.

So the second model is a statistical model using skills and drills. I am looking for a balance of capacity across training modalities.

The third model uses the three metabolic pathways. These are the three engines that produce adenosine triphosphate (ATP), the currency of effort of all energy output. Power is plotted on the Y-axis and duration of effort (time) on the X-axis. The first pathway (phosphagen or phosphocreatine) is high powered and short duration. It can account for about 100 percent of max human output and taps out at about 10 seconds. The second pathway (lactate or glycolytic) is moderate powered, moderate duration. It accounts for approximately 70 percent of max power output, peaks at about 60 seconds and terminates at 120 seconds. The third pathway (oxidative or aerobic) is low powered, long duration. It accounts for approximately 40 percent of max power output and does not fade in any reasonable time for which I have the patience to measure. The phosphagen and the glycolytic pathways are anaerobic; oxidative is aerobic. All three engines work all the time to some extent. The degree to which each is active is dependent on the activity. One idles, while the other two rev; two will rev, one will idle, etc.

Our thought is this: He or she is as fit as he or she is balanced in capacity in all three of these engines. A human being is a vehicle with three engines. Suppose we discover there is a fourth engine; we want capacity there, too. We develop capacity in all engines through our prescription: constantly varied functional movement executed at high intensity. We are looking for a balance in the bioenergetics (the engines that fuel all human activity).

DEFINITION OF FITNESS (2002-2008)
Although clumsy, these three models served as a litmus test for the fitness we were after. And we moved forward. We launched CrossFit.com and posted the Workout of the Day (WOD): constantly varied, high-intensity functional movement.

We were collecting the data from doing WODs and started asking: "What does it really mean to do Fran? What does it really mean to do Helen? What does it mean to say that your time went from 7 minutes to 6 minutes to 5 minutes to 4 minutes?" Some interesting things came of this.

The workout Fran is 21-15-9 thrusters (95 lb.) and pull-ups. Complete the workout by doing 21 thrusters (front squat 95 lb., then drive it overhead), then 21 pull-

TABLE 1. EXAMPLE WORK AND POWER CALCULATIONS BETWEEN BENCHMARK ATTEMPTS	
Workout	Fran 21-15-9 Thrusters, 95 lb. Pull-ups

Athlete	6 ft. tall 200 lb.

Work	**Per Rep**	**Force** x	**Distance** =	**Work (approx.)**
	Pull-up	200 lb.	24 in. x $\frac{1\ ft.}{12\ in.}$	400 ft.-lb.
	Thruster (athlete)	200 lb.	26 in. x $\frac{1\ ft.}{12\ in.}$	433 ft.-lb.
	Thruster (barbell)	95 lb.	47 in. x $\frac{1\ ft.}{12\ in.}$	372 ft.-lb.
			TOTAL	1,205 ft.-lb.
	Per Fran	**Reps** x	**Work** =	**Total (approx.)**
		45	1,205 ft.-lb.	54,225 ft.-lb.

Power	**Date**	**Finished Time**	**Power Output (approx.)**
	April 2015	4 min. 30 sec.	54,225 ft.-lb. / 4.5 min. = 12,050 ft.-lb. / min.
	May 2016	2 min. 45 sec.	54,225 ft.-lb. / 2.75 min. = 19,718 ft.-lb. / min.

Change in Power		**April 2015**	**May 2016**	**Change (approx.)**
	Power	12,050 ft.-lb. / min. vs.	19,718 ft.-lb. / min.	60% increase in power
	Time	4.5 min. vs.	2.75 min.	60% decrease in time
	Conclusion	Time approximates our change in power output.		

ups (get your chin over a bar from a hang anyhow). Then go back to the thrusters for 15 repetitions, 15 pull-ups, 9 of each, stop the clock, and we get a total time for the effort.

Power is force times distance (work) divided by time. The work required to do Fran is constant (force times distance). It does not change unless your height changes (distance), the distance we travel (the movement's range of motion) changes, the load changes (95 lb.), or your weight changes. This means that every time you do Fran or a specific benchmark workout, the work is constant.

So, you do Fran for the first time and have a Time 1 for it (T1). If you do it a year later, the same work was completed but you have a separate time (T2). In comparing the two efforts, we find that the work quantity cancels and the difference in time is the difference in power produced (Table 1).

There will be measurement error in this calculation. I can measure the force/weight with a scale, the distance traveled with a tape measure, and time with a watch. There is not a lot of error therein, but there are some concerns as we are calculating the body's displacement by using the center of mass, for example. However, as long as the work is constant, the same error occurs with every effort. And in comparison from one effort to the next, the errors cancel each other out (zero order error). This ratio of time (T2/T1) describes my progress to the accuracy and precision of the watch, which is the best of my three tools (stopwatch, tape measure, scale).

By tracking the difference in time between workout attempts, we are looking at changes in power. We did not have to study this much longer to come to this understanding that your collection of workout data points represented your work capacity across broad time and modal domains. This is your fitness.

With power on the Y-axis and duration of effort on the X-axis, the power output of any effort can be plotted. Take a handful of efforts that take approximately 10 seconds to do, measure their power output individually, and then get an average of these efforts. Repeat this exercise at 30 seconds, 2 minutes, 10 minutes, 60 minutes, etc. Plot these data points. With adequate scientific accuracy and precision, I have graphed mathematically an individual's work capacity across broad time and modal domains (Figure 1).

A FOURTH MODEL AND THE DEFINITION OF HEALTH (2008)

Along the way in using these three models, we had also observed that there was a continuum of measures from sickness to wellness to fitness. If it was a measure I could quantify, something of interest to a physician or exercise physiologist, we find it would sit well ordered on this pattern.

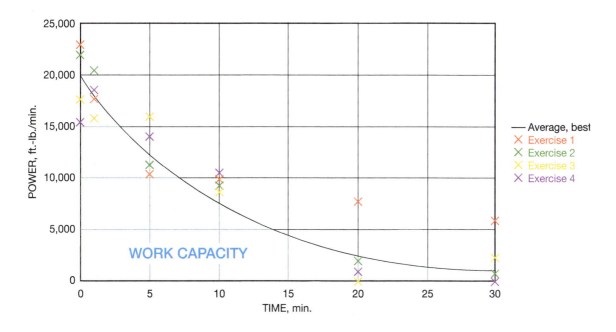

Figure 1. A Graphical Representation of One's Fitness (Work Capacity)
at a Certain Time in His or Her Life.

Take body fat, for example. If you are 40 percent body fat, that is considered mor-
bidly obese. The numbers vary by community, but 15 percent is often considered
well or normal. Five percent is typically what you would see in an elite athlete. Bone
density follows a similar pattern. There is a level of bone density that is pathological; it is osteoporosis or osteopenia in early stages. There is a value that is normal.
We find gymnasts with three to five times normal bone density. I can do this with
a resting heart rate, flexibility (any of the 10 general physical skills), and even some
subjective things to which we cannot put numbers through analytical methods
(e.g., mood). I do not know of a metric that runs counter to this pattern. This observation led us to believe that fitness and health were varying different measures of
the same reality.

This also means that if you are fit, you first have to become well to become patho-
logically sick. It tells me that fitness is a hedge against sickness, with wellness as
an intermediate value.

If there is anything in your lifestyle, training regimen or recreational pursuits that
has one of these metrics moving in a wrong direction, I want you to entertain the
possibility you are doing something profoundly wrong. What we find is when you
do CrossFit (constantly varied, high-intensity functional movements), eat meat
and vegetables, nuts and seeds, some fruit, little starch, no sugar, and get plenty of
sleep every night, we do not have this divergent side effect. It does not work such

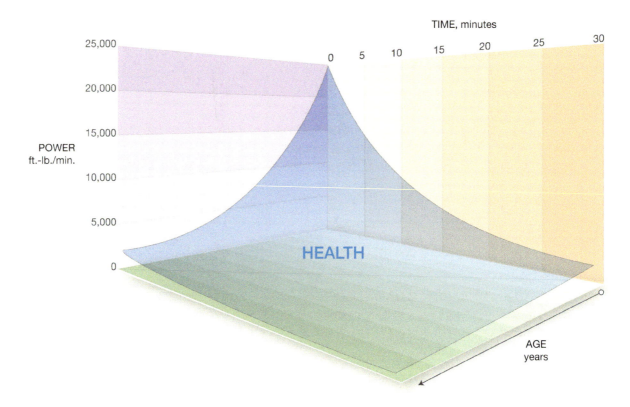

Figure 2. A Graphical Representation of One's Health
(Fitness Throughout His or Her Life).

that everything is improving except one value. We knew this observation could be another test in assessing one's fitness regimen.

Recall that we represent fitness as the area under the curve on a graph with power on the Y-axis and duration of effort on the X-axis. By adding a third dimension, age, on the Z-axis and extending the fitness across, it produces a three-dimensional solid (Figure 2). That is health. And with this measure, I have the same relationship to things that seemingly matter: high-density lipoproteins (HDL), triglycerides, heart rate, anything that the doctor would tell you is important.

I am of the opinion that health would be maximally held by maximizing your area under the curve and holding that work capacity for as long as you can. In other words: Eat meat and vegetables, nuts and seeds, some fruit, little starch, no sugar; do constantly varied high-intensity exercise; learn and play new sports throughout your life. This will buy you more health than will trying to fix your cholesterol or bone density with a pharmaceutical intervention. That it is a failed approach.

I want you to understand how these definitions of fitness and health are different than those found in exercise-science literature. First, understand that our definitions of these quantities are measurable. One of the problems with exercise science is that it would very rarely meet the rigors of any real science (chemistry, physics, engineering).

Secondly, it is also almost never about exercise. For example, maximal oxygen consumption (VO_2 max) and lactate threshold are correlates, maybe components, but absolutely subordinate to what happens to work capacity. Who would take an increase in VO_2 max for a decrease in work capacity across broad time and modal domains? What that would look like is breathing more air than you ever had before on a treadmill test in a lab but losing the road race. Similarly, someone's lactate threshold could increase, but he or she still gets choked out in the fight because of lack of work capacity.

I could make a list of hundreds of these metrics, and no one has ever produced a great athlete by advancing them one at a time. It does not happen. I can move them best by doing constantly varied, high-intensity functional movements; doing things that look like Fran, Diane, Helen; turning fitness into sport by working with fixed workloads and trying to minimize the time by making every workout a competitive effort among the cohort. And when I do that, what we find is that these metrics do spectacular things.

Suppose a man at 90 years old is living independently, running up and down the steps and playing with his grandchildren. We would not be concerned if his cholesterol numbers were "high." There is a problem looking only at longevity. Imagine a curve that stretches to 90 or even 105 years but has very low work capacity for its duration. That is not what CrossFit is about: It is about vitality and capacity. What can you do?

It is imperative for making meaningful assertions about training that fitness and health are measurable. The area (or volume) under the curve gives me a scientifically accurate, precise and valid measure of an athlete's fitness (or health). And we are the first to have ever done that. When we showed this to physicists, chemists, engineers, they agreed there is no other way to assess the capacity of something, be it a rocket, motorcycle, truck or human. Tell me how much it weighs, how far it moves and how long it takes. Everything else is entirely irrelevant. ▪

Learn the mechanics of fundamental movements, establish a consistent pattern of practicing these same movements, and, only then, ratchet up the intensity of workouts incorporating these movements. 'Mechanics,' then 'Consistency,' and then 'Intensity'– this is the key to effective implementation of CrossFit programming."

–COACH GLASSMAN

TECHNIQUE

Adapted from Coach Glassman's Dec. 1, 2007, L1 lecture in Charlotte, North Carolina.

In no small part, what is behind this program is the quantification of fitness. This means we put a number on fitness: work capacity across broad time and modal domains. You can assess one's fitness by determining the area under his or her work-capacity curve. This would be similar to a group of athletes competing in 25 to 30 workouts. Include a range of activities—like three pulls on the Concept2 rower for average watts to a 10-mile run—and a multitude of workouts in between. Compile their overall placing across these events, and everyone then has a reasonable metric of his or her total capacity.

This quantification of fitness is a part of a broader concept that is at the heart of this movement: We call it evidence-based fitness. This means measurable, observable, repeatable data is used in analyzing and assessing a fitness program. There are three meaningful components to analysis of a fitness program: safety, efficacy, and efficiency.

The efficacy of a program means, "What is the return?" Maybe a fitness program advertises that it will make you a better soccer player. There needs to be evidence of this supported by measurable, observable, repeatable data. For CrossFit, we want to increase your work capacity across broad time and modal domains. This is the efficacy of this program. What are the tangible results? What is the adaptation that the program induces?

Efficiency is the time rate of that adaptation. Maybe the fitness program advertises that it can deliver 50 pull-ups. There is a big difference whether it takes six months versus nine years to achieve that.

Safety is how many people end up at the finish line. Suppose I have a fitness program. I start with 10 individuals: Two of them become the fittest human beings on Earth and the other eight die. While I would rather be one of the two fittest than the eight dead, and I do not know if I want to play, I am not going to attach a normative value to it. The real tragedy comes in not knowing the safety numbers.

These three vectors of safety, efficacy and efficiency point in the same direction, such that they are not entirely at odds with each other. I can greatly increase the safety of a program by turning the efficacy and efficiency down to zero. I can increase the efficiency by turning up the intensity and then possibly compromising safety. Or I could damage the efficacy by losing people. Safety, efficacy and efficiency are the three meaningful aspects of a program. They give me all I need to assess it.

This quantification of fitness, by choosing work capacity as our standard for the efficacy of the program, necessitates the qualification of movement. Our quantification of fitness introduces qualification of movement.

For the qualification of movement there are four common terms: mechanics, technique, form and style. I will not delve into them with too much detail: The distinction is not that important. I use both technique and form somewhat interchangeably, although there is a slightly nuanced distinction.

When I talk about angular velocity, momentum, leverage, origin or insertion of muscles, torque, force, power, relative angles, we are taking about mechanics. When I speak to the physics of movement, and especially the statics and less so the dynamics, I am looking at the mechanics.

Technique is the method to success for completion of a movement. For example, if you want to do a full twisting dismount on the rings, the technique would be: pull, let go, look, arm up, turn, shoulder drop, etc. Technique includes head posture and body posture. And there are effective and less effective techniques. Technique includes the mechanics, but it is in the macro sense of "how do you complete the movement without the physics?"

Form is the normative value: This is good or this is bad—"you should" or "you shouldn't" applied to mechanics and technique.

Style is essentially the signature to a movement; that is, that aspect of the movement that is fairly unique to you. The best of the weightlifting coaches can look at the bar path during a lift and tell you which lifter it is. There are aspects to all of our movements that define us like your thumbprint. It is the signature. To be truly just the signature, style elements have no bearing on form, technique or mechanics. Style does not enter into the normative assessment, is not important to technique, and does not alter substantially the physics.

These four terms are all qualifications to movement. I want to speak generally to technique and form to include all of this, but what we are talking about here is the non-quantification of output; that is, how you move.

By taking power or work capacity as our primary value for assessing technique—and this reliance on functional movement—we end up in kind of an interesting position. We end up where power is the successful completion of functional movement.

This is not about merely energy exerted. On a graph, you could put work completed on the X-axis and energy expended on the Y-axis. Someone could potentially expend a lot of energy and do very little work by being inefficient. Ideally, what that individual would do would see little energy expended for the maximum amount of work. Technique is what maximizes the work completed for the energy expended (Figure 1). For any given capacity, say metabolically, for energy expenditure, the guy who knows the technique is going to be able to do the most amount of work.

Suppose I take two people at random and they are both trying the same task. One is familiar with how to deadlift, and one is not. One knows how to clean, one does

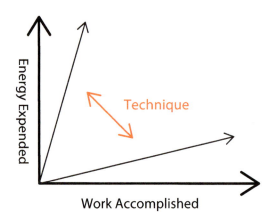

Figure 1. Technique Maximizes the Work Accomplished for the Energy Expended.

not. One knows how to drive overhead, one does not. Suppose they are loading a truck with sandbags. The one familiar with lifting large objects and transporting them is going to do a lot more work.

You can have the argument as to who is stronger. For example, you can use an electromyogram and see with what force the biceps shortens. If you are defining strength as contractile potential, you may end up with the guy with enormous contractile potential—but not knowing the technique of the clean, the jerk, the deadlift, he cannot do as much work.

We, however, do not take contractile potential as the gold standard for strength. Strength is the productive application of force. If you cannot complete work, if you cannot express strength as power, if strength cannot be expressed as productive result, it does not count. Having enormous biceps and quadriceps is useless if you cannot run, jump, lift, throw, press.

This is related to safety, efficacy and efficiency because technique (quality of movement) is the heart of maximizing each of these.

He or she who knows how to do these movements when confronted with them will get a better result in terms of safety. Two individuals attempt to lift a heavy object; one knows how to pop a hip and get under it (clean), and the other guy starts to pull with a rounded back. I can tell you what is likely to happen to he or she who does not know how to lift. If you want to stay safe, you better have good technique, good form.

Efficacy, for any given contractile potential, for any given limit to your total metabolic capacity, he or she who knows the technique will be able to get more work done and will develop faster. If after six months of teaching you how to clean it still does not look like I would like it to, you will not get twice body weight overhead more quickly than someone who looks like a natural. You want an effective program, you are going to have to move with quality, you want to get the result quickly—technique is going to be pivotal to your success.

Technique is an intimate part of safety, efficacy, and efficiency.

We can see how this manifests in CrossFit workouts by way of a comparison. I want to look at typing, shooting, playing the violin, NASCAR driving and CrossFit. What these domains have in common is that a marked proficiency is associated with speed. Being able to shoot accurately and quickly is better than quickly or accurately.

You may try to get a job as a typist because you do not make any mistakes. However, for this perfection, you type at a rate of 20 words a minute and only use two fingers. You will never get hired. Playing the violin fast and error-free is critical for a virtuoso. However, someone who gets through "Flight of the Bumblebee" in 12 minutes is not there yet. A NASCAR driver wants to both drive fast and not wreck. In CrossFit, a perfectly exquisite Fran is worthless if it takes 32 minutes.

And yet, it is presented to CrossFit coaches as, "Should I use good form or should I do it quickly?" I do not like my choices. One is impossible without the other.

Technique and speed are not at odds with one another, where "speed" is related to all the quantification of the movement: power, force, distance, time. They are seemingly at odds. It is a misapprehension. It is an illusion.

Can you learn to drive fast without wrecking? Can you learn to type fast without making errors? Can you shoot quickly without missing? Eventually, but not in the learning. One is impossible without the other.

You will not learn to type fast without typing where you make a ton of errors and then work to reduce the errors at that speed. Then you go faster, and then again pull the errors back in, then go faster and pull the errors back in. You drive faster and faster and then you spin out in the infield or you hit the wall.

If you are a race driver and you have never spun out, gone out in the infield or never been in a wreck, you are not very good. If you are a typist and you have never made a mistake, you are very slow. In CrossFit, if your technique is perfect, your intensity is always low.

Here is the part that is hard to understand: You will not maximize the intensity or the speed without mistakes. But it is not the mistakes that make you faster. It is not reaching for the letter P with your pinky and hitting the O. It is not hitting the wrong note that made you play faster. It is not missing the target by two feet that made you a better shooter. It is not running into the wall that made you a faster driver. But you will not get there without it. The errors are an unavoidable consequence of development.

This iterative process of letting this scope of errors broaden then reducing them without reducing the speed is called "threshold training."

In a CrossFit workout, if you are moving well, I will tell you to pick up the speed. Suppose at the higher speed the movement still looks good: I will encourage you to go faster. And if it still looks good I will encourage you to go even faster. Now the movement starts falling apart.

I do not want you to slow down yet. First, at that speed I want you to fix your technique. What you need to do is continuously and constantly advance the margins at which form falters.

It may be that initially at 10,000 foot-pounds per minute my technique is perfect, but it falls apart at 12,000 foot-pounds per minute. Work at that 10,000 to 12,000 foot-pounds per minute mark to fix the form, and soon enough you will have great technique at 12,000 foot-pounds per minute. The next step is to achieve that technique at 14,000 foot-pounds per minute.

At first, the technique at 14,000 foot-pounds per minute will suffer. Then you must narrow it in. That is the process. It is ineluctable. It is unavoidable. There is nothing I can do about it. That is not my rule.

We are the technique people. We drill technique incessantly, but simultaneously I want you to go faster. You will learn to work at higher intensity with good technique only by ratcheting up the intensity to a point where good technique is impossible. This dichotomy means that it is impossible at the limits of your capacity to obey every little detail and nuance of technique. Some of the refined motor-recruitment patterns are not going to always look perfect.

I do not know of a domain where speed matters and technique is not at the heart of it. In every athletic endeavor where we can quantify the output, there is incredible technique at the highest levels of performance.

Suppose someone set the new world record for the shot put, but his technique was poor. This means one of two things: one, either with good technique it would have gone farther, or two, we were wrong in understanding what is good technique.

Technique is everything. It is at the heart of our quantification. You will not express power in significant measure without technique. You might expend a lot of energy, but you will not see the productive application of force. You will not be able to complete functional tasks efficiently or effectively. You will not be safe in trying.

There is a perceived paradox here that really is not a paradox when you understand the factors at play. ▪

NUTRITION: AVOIDING DISEASE AND OPTIMIZING PERFORMANCE

Adapted from Coach Glassman's Sept. 9, 2007, L1 lecture in Quantico, Virginia, and Oct. 14, 2007, L1 lecture in Flagstaff, Arizona.

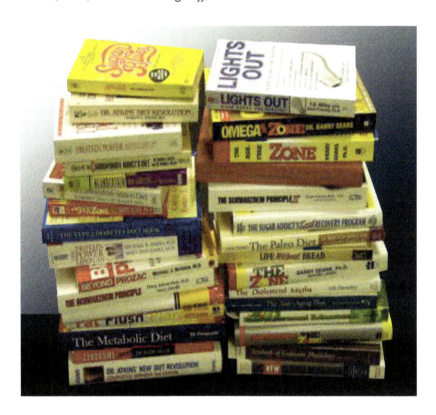

The CrossFit message is contrarian. It is against the grain of what occurs at most commercial gyms. They have machines; we detest them. They use isolation movements; we use compound movements. They use low intensity; we use high intensity. Everything about this message is for many people antithetical to all they thought they knew. With nutrition, the theme continues: What most everyone thinks is wrong.

In July of 1989 in the Archives of Internal Medicine, Norman Kaplan wrote an absolutely breathtaking bit of research. It is an analysis that has gone completely unchallenged. He was able to demonstrate by an operative mechanism, through correlation, and more importantly causally, that hyperinsulinism is at the root of the "deadly quartet" (i.e., upper-body obesity, glucose intolerance, hypertriglyceridemia and hypertension). Hyperinsulinism—too much insulin—was the cause.

If you are healthy, insulin is the normal and essential response to the ingestion of carbohydrate. Insulin is a hormone produced by the pancreas, and you cannot live without it. You can either produce insulin through the pancreas, you can inject it, or you can die. Insulin is responsible for storage of energy in cells. (Glucagon is the counter-regulatory hormone to insulin: It releases the energy out of the cells.) And one of the things that insulin puts into cells is fat.

You can see that the way to get your insulin level too high (hyperinsulinism) is to eat too much carbohydrate. How much carbohydrate is that? In the qualitative sense, your insulin level is "too high" if it is driving up your blood pressure, making you fat or reducing your ability to suppress blood sugar after eating carbohydrate. If you are glucose intolerant, hypertensive or your triglycerides are too high, you are getting too much insulin and thus too much carbohydrate. These are risk factors for heart disease, and the process by which we induce atherosclerotic disease—arteries paved over with plaque. This leads to thrombosis, occlusion, myocardial infarct and debilitation and death. But when physicians are polled "what is it that you do not want to get?" cancer and heart disease do not rate nearly so high as does Type 2 diabetes.

And I can tell you how to get it. Type 2 diabetes is caused by a receptor downgrade phenomenon on the liver, muscle, and fat cells. They have a receptor site where insulin attaches. It is similar to a key fitting in a lock—specific shapes on each allow them to bind together. When insulin binds to the receptor, the cell can now receive all good things, including amino acids (proteins) and fat.

If you expose yourself to too much insulin, the cells and receptors become "blind" to it. The key does not work as well in the lock; i.e., receptor downgrade phenomenon. The mechanism is not really much different mechanically than staring at the sun. At first, your eyes see light, but if you do it for a few minutes, you will never see any light again. You just burned out the receptors. That is what happens in Type 2 diabetes.

What was revolutionary about Kaplan's work is that it disproved an accepted model. Traditionally, what was observed over tens of years was that individuals often first gained weight (obesity), then their cholesterol went up (hypercholesterolemia), then their blood pressure went up (hypertensive), and then they become diabetic. There was an assumption—and it is a classical logical fallacy—that the ordering suggested causality. That because this happened first, then this—it was the root cause of all the other conditions. This model is now understood to be fatally flawed (i.e., a post hoc, ergo propter hoc fallacy). Order of events does not necessitate causality.

Kaplan was able to demonstrate with powerful evidence that hyperinsulinism was the cause of all these conditions, the cause of atherosclerotic disease and cardiac death. All of this is collectively known as coronary heart disease (CHD).

There has been a very powerful shift and re-understanding that what is causing heart disease is not dietary-fat intake but excessive consumption of carbohydrate. Things like the French paradox show that there is no paradox. The paradigm was flawed. The French eat many times the fat that Americans do and yet have a much smaller frequency of heart disease. They also consume just a little bit under 5 percent of the refined sugar we do. We are eating about 150 lb. of sugar per man, woman, and child annually.

It is amazing what efforts we will exert to consume sugar. Your interest in carbohydrates, and it is profound, is really no different than your interest in beer or opiates. Sugar tickles the brain and it feels good. And the excuses and things people will do to get to that high are unbelievable.

Now I tell you how to avoid all of that.

Eat a diet of meat and vegetables, nuts and seeds, some fruit, little starch and no sugar.

Do that and you are exempt.

Meat and vegetables, nuts and seeds, some fruit, little starch, no sugar—and no coronary heart disease.

It has nothing to do with genetics. The genetic part is an intolerance to excess amounts of carbohydrate. It is no different than having a genetic predisposition to alcoholism. Having the gene for alcoholism does not mean it will necessarily be expressed. You would have to drink alcohol. If you do not drink alcohol, you probably will not suffer from alcoholism, at least not in the clinical manifestation of it.

It is no different with atherosclerotic disease. I do not care what your grandfather died of, your mother died of, your uncle died of, your brother died of. For example, Dr. Barry Sears, all his uncles and father died at 49 years old from atherosclerotic-induced thrombosis, myocardial infarct, heart attack. All of them. He is not going to. He is not eating the carbohydrates they ate.

Eat meat and vegetables, nuts and seeds, some fruit, little starch, no sugar. To get to the same endpoint, these are effective nutritional strategies for avoiding heart disease, death and misery:

1) If you could not have harvested it out of your garden or farm and eaten it an hour later, it is not food.

2) Shop around the perimeter of the grocery store, and do not go down the aisles.

3) If it has a food label on it, it is not food. You do not see that on the chicken. It is not on the tomatoes. But it is on the chips and cookies.

4) If it is not perishable, if it says "Best if used before 2019," it is not food.

In 1995, we were delivering almost the same lecture with just less clinical experience. And people were like: "You are kidding me?" and "Fat makes you fat, right?" It is not true.

OPTIMIZING PERFORMANCE

The next layer to diet is about optimizing performance. Through a diet of meat and vegetables, nuts and seeds, some fruit, little starch, no sugar, you will not be so lucky as to optimize your output. To get a sub-three-minute Fran, you need to weigh and measure your meat and vegetables, nuts and seeds, fruit and starch, and you need to eliminate sugar.

I wish it were not true. I wish the path of fitness was riding bicycles and drinking beer. I wished that is how we did it. It does not work. What you have to do is eat meat and vegetables, nuts and seeds, some fruit, little starch, no sugar, and then get a scale and measuring cup. You need accuracy and precision to your consumption or you will never get in a jet stream of elite performance.

If you want to have top-fuel-type performance, you need top fuel. I wish it were otherwise. What do I base this on? No one has ever demonstrated to me anything but inferior capacity on a diet where they did not weigh and measure.

I am not telling you that you have to weigh and measure your food. But I am telling you that you are not going to get anywhere in terms of optimizing your performance on a bad diet. And we have seen enough incidences now. I have worked with tens of thousands of people: No one has ever done it.

You need to weigh and measure your food. Not forever, but at least to start. It is also good to go back to weighing and measuring once in a while. What happens is that the portion requirements diminish for all the foods you do not like. "Yes, I only need one spear of asparagus. Ice cream? I think it was a pound." You will bias in the wrong direction.

I can take any cohort, get one of them to weigh and measure food, and he or she will pull away. There are very few things you can do short of doing more pull-ups that can get you more pull-ups other than eating the way we recommend it. There is a one-to-one correspondence between elite CrossFit performance and the accuracy and precision of their consumption.

And what you are going to find is performance improvement after performance improvement, but at some point you will want to stop the athlete from leaning out further. It is possible you will get too lean to perform well. You may find a plateau in your output, and then you need to ratchet it up. (I do the same thing for hard gainers; I increase their intake as I do not need them to lean out.) The first step: When you get as lean as you want to be and before there is a diminution in performance, double the fat. If you do not feel a whole lot better, maybe try three times the fat. And if that does not feel a whole lot better, and instead you just get thicker, then go back to two times the fat. But I would let performance tell me what to do. In making modifications, I want to see any kind of change in physiognomy. I have more room to play with when someone has extra padding; I have to be more careful with someone who is already ripped.

The formula for calculating what is relevant and pertinent to your prescription is lean body mass and activity level. Done. There is not an inherent difference for men versus women, for young versus old. I want to know how active you are and I want to know what your lean body mass is. And everything else is not germane, not pertinent, not relevant. It is extraneous information.

In the vagaries and contingencies of everyday living, such as schedules and appetite, there are fluctuations in intake that will occur without weighing and measuring. Following these normal fluctuations puts you on a coarser path versus the fine path required for optimized performance. And that is why you will not get there by luck. It is also possible an average CrossFit athlete becomes extraordinary this way. Commitment and focus are going to overcome genetic limitations. If you commit to the effort, you stand a much better chance. We have had this fantastic experience of playing with this. In any cohort, one pulls away when he or she is weighing and measuring food in this 40-30-30 milieu of macronutrient intake. ▪

FITNESS, LUCK AND HEALTH

Adapted from Coach Glassman's Feb. 27, 2016, L1 lecture in San Jose, California; March 27, 2016, L1 lecture in Aromas, California; and April 24, 2016, L1 lecture in Oakland, California.

In 2002, we observed that almost any health parameter sits well ordered on a continuum of values that ranged from sick to well to fit. High-density lipoproteins (HDL cholesterol), for instance: At less than 35 mg/dL you have a problem, 50 mg/dL is nice, and 75 mg/dL is a whole lot better. Blood pressure: 195/115 mm/Hg you have a problem, 120/70 mm/Hg is healthy, and 105/50 mm/Hg looks more like an athlete. Triglycerides, bone density, muscle mass, body fat, hemoglobin A1c (HbA1c, aka glycated hemoglobin)—all can be plotted relative to these three values.

The significance is that these are the predictors, the cause, and the manifestation of chronic disease. Chronic diseases include obesity, coronary heart disease, Type 2 diabetes, stroke, cancer (to include breast, colon and lung, but my theory is this will include all the positron-emission-tomography-positive cancers eventually, which are 95 percent of all cancers), Alzheimer's, peripheral artery disease, advanced biological aging, drug addiction, among others.

It is very likely that if you have any chronic disease, you have deranged markers. If you have Alzheimer's, you would see your HDL suppressed, your blood pressure up, your triglycerides up, your body fat up, your muscle mass down, your bone density down, your HbA1c high, etc. The same is true with diabetes. The same is true with most cancers.

Medicine has no effective treatment for chronic disease: It is symptomatic only. The doctor gives you a drug to bring your cholesterol down, a different drug to raise your bone density. You might need bariatric surgery if you have morbid obesity. If you have paved-over coronary arteries, they can do bypass surgery. If you become glucose intolerant, the doctor can put you on insulin. But all of these are not fixes. They are masking the problem. If you have persistent malignant hypertension, you should take an antihypertensive if you cannot get your blood pressure down otherwise. But how would you get it down otherwise?

CrossFit, Inc. holds a uniquely elegant solution to the greatest problem facing the world today. It is not global warming or climate change. It is not the worst two choices imaginable for president. It is chronic disease. The CrossFit stimulus—which is constantly varied, high-intensity functional movement coupled with meat and vegetables, nuts and seeds, some fruit, little starch and no sugar—can give you a pass on chronic disease. It is elegant in the mathematical sense of being marked by simplicity and efficacy. It is so simple.

Seventy percent of deaths in the United States (U.S.) are attributable to chronic disease. Of the 2.6 million people who died in the U.S. in 2014, 1.8 million died from chronic disease. This pattern of increasing deaths due to chronic diseases also holds in countries that are ravaged by infectious disease. The numbers are rising, and when we finally add the positron-emission-tomography-positive cancers in, the number might be 80-85 percent in the U.S. It is estimated by the Centers for Disease Control (CDC) that the U.S. could have up to a hundred million diabetics in 2050. That will affect everyone. You will not go into the emergency room for something as simple as a broken arm: You will be seeing heart attacks on every corner. Medicine has no solution; you do. CrossFit, with meat and vegetables, nuts and seeds, some fruit, little starch and no sugar, will help you avoid all of this.

The other 30 percent are dying from accidents that come in four "-ic" variants: kinetic, genetic, toxic, and microbic. Kinetic: physical trauma, car crash, hit on a bike. Toxic: environmental toxins, such as lead poisoning. Genetic: genetic disorders like cystic fibrosis, you are born with it. Microbic: virus, bacteria, prions. This is where treatment can be symptomatic. This is where the miracles of medicine are. If you have got a genetic disorder that is making you sick, you need a doctor. If you have been poisoned, you need a doctor. If you caught a nasty virus or a flesh-eating bacteria, you need a doctor. You do not need to go to the gym, and you do not need burpees. Doctors are like lifeguards; CrossFit trainers are like swim coaches. When you are drowning, you do not need a swim coach. You needed one, and you did not get one. What you need is a lifeguard. We will teach people how to swim, and when they do not pay attention, and they go under, the doctors take care of it.

Accidents are largely stuff you can do nothing about, but there is one exception. Be fit. Kinetic: We hear stories from war of CrossFit athletes who survive things that people have not survived previously. Toxicity: Someone who is fitter is more likely to survive the same poisoning than someone who is not. Genetic: There are genes you have inherited that will or will not express because of your behavior through diet and exercise. Microbic: Who is most vulnerable to viral pneumonia? The frail, the feeble. So fitness offers a protection here.

But assume there is no protection from fitness because what you need in terms of preventing accidents largely is luck. Luck—there is no "good luck" versus "bad luck"—looks like not having these things happen to you. Seventy percent of what kills people can be addressed by what CrossFit trainers do, and the other 30 percent of deaths occur based on luck, so get fit and do not think about luck. If you stand around worried about germs, worried about the tire that is going to come through the windshield, worried about breathing toxic air, and worried about your genes, you are wasting your time. It will not make you happy. It will not make you better. It will not make you safer. You are not going to live any longer.

This sums to my "kinetic theory of health." The singular focus on kinematics—increasing work capacity, increasing your fitness—is how to avoid chronic disease. Just get a better Fran time, better deadlift, better Diane time, and do all the things that would support a better Fran time—like eating meat and vegetables, nuts and seeds, some fruit, little starch and no sugar; getting plenty of sleep; and maybe taking some fish oil. After that, we are out of stuff that matters. With that singular focus on work capacity, we can avoid chronic disease and there is nothing really to worry about. You have the lifestyle answer. Make it to the gym, eat like we tell you, and enjoy yourself. We have hacked health. Here is the magic formula for you:

Fitness + Luck (bad) = Health.

It is the part you can do something about plus the part you can do nothing about that sums to your outcome. So make the most out of fitness and you will not be part of the seven out of 10 who die unnecessarily due to lifestyle. In the end, chronic disease is a deficiency syndrome. It is sedentation with malnutrition.

The cost of chronic disease is such that U.S. medical expenditure is now about $4 trillion a year. In 2008, Pricewaterhousecoopers estimated that roughly half of all U.S. medical expenditure was wasted on unnecessary procedures, administrative inefficiencies, treatment of preventable conditions and so on. Add in fraud and abuse and we are wasting well more than a trillion dollars. We also know 86 percent of overall health-care spending goes to treating the chronically diseased ineffectively. Of the remaining 14 percent, half goes to the stuff that medicine can actually do something about. That means seven percent of health-care spending is not wasted. The amount spent on chronic disease is a waste.

What CrossFit trainers are providing is non-medical health care. When doctors treat those affected by accidents (the 30 percent), that is medical health care. If you are confused about the two, it is easy to distinguish by methods and tools. If someone is cut open, given radiation, prescribed pills, injected with syringes, it is medicine. It is treatment by a doctor.

On our side, it looks like CrossFit. We have rings, dumbbells, pull-up bars, our own bodies—and the prescription is universal. It is not to treat disease. It does not matter where you fall on this continuum: You get put on the same program. If the prescription is universal, it cannot be medicine. If it is something everyone needs—like air or oxygen—that is not medicine. Without vitamin C, you can get scurvy. Should physicians control orange and lemon groves, onion and kale production because they have vitamin C that you cannot live without? We do not want them doing that to food. We cannot let them do that to exercise, and there is a powerful movement with a lot of funding afoot to do exactly that. Millions of dollars are being spent to bring exercise into the purview of the medical arena so that it falls under the Affordable Care Act.

We have 13,000 gyms with 2 to 4 million people safe from chronic disease right now. This community is doing a lot of good things on a lot of fronts. Yet our gyms are thriving not because of our impact on chronic disease. They are thriving because the end users, the customers, are extremely happy with the transformation. And it is part physical, part emotional, part health markers, part relationships. That is the miracle of CrossFit: People are getting something that they did not even know they wanted or needed. ∎

ZONE MEAL PLANS

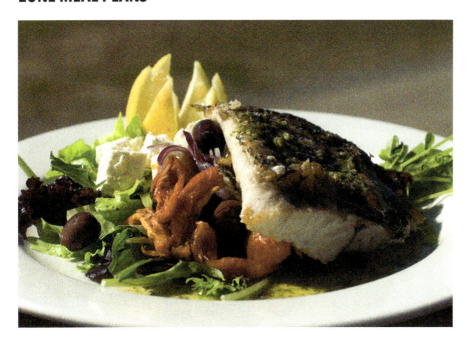

Originally published in May 2004.

Our recommendation to "eat meat and vegetables, nuts and seeds, some fruit, little starch, and no sugar" is adequate to the task of preventing the scourges of diet-induced disease, but a more accurate and precise prescription is necessary to optimize physical performance.

Finely tuned, a good diet will increase energy, sense of well-being, and acumen, while simultaneously flensing fat and packing on muscle. When properly composed, the right diet can nudge every important quantifiable marker for health in the right direction.

Diet is critical to optimizing human function, and our clinical experience leads us to believe that Dr. Barry Sears' Zone Diet closely models optimal nutrition.

CrossFit's best performers are Zone eaters. When our second-tier athletes commit to strict adherence to the Zone parameters, they generally become top-tier performers quickly. It seems that the Zone Diet accelerates and amplifies the effects of the CrossFit regimen.

Unfortunately, the full benefit of the Zone Diet is largely limited to those who have at least at first weighed and measured their food.

For a decade, we experimented with sizing and portioning strategies that avoid scales, and measuring cups and spoons, only to conclude that natural variances in caloric intake and macronutrient composition without measurement are greater than the resolution required to turn good performance to great. Life would be much easier for us were this not so!

The 1-Block Equivalents for Protein, Fat, and Carbohydrates (Figure 1, Table 3) and Sample Zone Meals and Snacks (Table 4) have been our most expedient approach for eliciting athletes' best performances and optimal health.

Even discounting any theoretical or technical content, this portal to sound nutrition still requires some basic arithmetic and weighing and measuring portions for the first weeks.

Too many athletes, after supposedly reading Sears' book "Enter the Zone," still ask, "So what do I eat for dinner?" They get meal plans and block charts. We can make the Zone more complicated or simpler, but not more effective.

We encourage everyone to weigh and measure portions for a couple weeks because it is supremely worth the effort, not because it is fun. If you choose to "guesstimate" portions, you will have the result of CrossFit's top performers only if and when you are lucky.

Within a couple of weeks of weighing and measuring, you will have developed an uncanny ability to estimate the mass of common food portions, but, more importantly, you will have formed a keen visual sense of your nutritional needs. This is a profound awareness.

In the Zone scheme, all of humanity calculates to either 2-, 3-, 4-, or 5-block meals at breakfast, lunch, and dinner, with either 1- or 2-block snacks between lunch and dinner and again between dinner and bedtime. We have simplified the process for determining which of the four meal sizes and two snack sizes best suits your needs (Table 1). We assume that you are doing CrossFit; i.e., active.

Being a "4-blocker," for instance, means that you eat three meals each day, where each meal is composed of 4 blocks of protein, 4 blocks of carbohydrate, and 4 blocks of fat. Whether you are a "smallish" medium-sized guy or a "largish" medium-sized guy would determine whether you will need snacks of 1 or 2 blocks twice a day (Table 2).

The "meal plans" we give stand as examples of 2-, 3-, 4-, or 5-block meals, and the "block chart" gives quantities of common foods equivalent to 1 block of protein, carbohydrate, or fat.

Once you determine that you need, say, 4-block meals, it is simple to use the block chart and select four times something from the protein list, four times something from the carbohydrate list, and four times something from the fat list every meal.

One-block snacks are chosen from the block chart at face value for a single snack of protein, carbohydrate, and fat, whereas 2-block snacks are, naturally, composed of twice something from the carbohydrate list combined with twice something from the protein list and twice something from the fat list.

Every meal, every snack, must contain equivalent blocks of protein, carbohydrate, and fat.

If the protein source is specifically labeled "non-fat," then double the usual fat blocks for that meal. Read "Enter the Zone" to learn why.

For those eating according to Zone parameters, body fat comes off fast. When our men fall below 10 percent body fat and start approaching 5 percent, we kick up the fat intake. The majority of our best athletes end up at X blocks of protein, X blocks of carbohydrate, and 4X or 5X blocks of fat. Learn to modulate fat intake to produce a level of leanness that optimizes performance.

The Zone Diet neither prohibits nor requires any particular food. It can accommodate paleo or vegan, organic or kosher, fast food or fine dining, while delivering the benefits of high-performance nutrition. ▪

A block is a unit of measure used to simplify the process of making balanced meals.

- 7 g of protein = 1 block of protein
- 9 g of carbohydrate = 1 block of carbohydrate
- 3 g of fat = 1 block of fat

Because most protein sources contain fat (e.g., meat), individuals should only add 1.5 g for each fat block when constructing meals. The block chart on the following pages outlines an amount of each item to achieve 1.5 g of fat.

When a meal is composed of equal blocks of protein, carbohydrate, and fat, 40 percent of its calories are from carbohydrate, 30 percent from protein and 30 percent from fat.

The following pages contain common foods in their macronutrient category (protein, carbohydrate, or fat), along with a conversion of measurements to a block.

This "block chart" of 1-block equivalents is a convenient tool for making balanced meals. Simply choose 1 item from the protein list, 1 item from the carbohydrate list, and 1 item from the fat list to compose a 1-block meal. Or choose 2 items from each column to compose a 2-block meal, and so on.

Here is a sample 4-block meal:

- 4 oz. chicken breast
- 1 artichoke
- 1 cup of steamed vegetables with 24 crushed peanuts
- 1 sliced apple

This meals contains 28 g of protein, 36 g of carbohydrate, and 12 g of fat. It is simpler, though, to think of it as a 4-block meal.

Figure 1. Block Composition.

TABLE 1. BLOCK PRESCRIPTION BASED ON SEX AND BODY TYPE

Body Type	Breakfast	Lunch	Snack	Dinner	Snack	Total Blocks
Small female	2	2	2	2	2	10
Medium female	3	3	1	3	1	11
Large female	3	3	2	3	2	13
Athletic, well-muscled female	4	4	1	4	1	14
Small male	4	4	2	4	2	16
Medium male	5	5	1	5	1	17
Large male	5	5	2	5	2	19
Extra-large male	4	4	4	4	4	20
Hard gainer	5	5	3	5	3	21
Large hard gainer	5	5	4	5	4	23
Athletic, well-muscled male	5	5	5	5	5	25

TABLE 2. SAMPLE 1-DAY BLOCK REQUIREMENTS FOR SMALL (16-BLOCK) MALE

	Breakfast	Lunch	Snack	Dinner	Snack
Protein	4	4	2	4	2
Carbohydrate	4	4	2	4	2
Fat	4	4	2	4	2

PROTEINS			
Food	Eyeball	Exact Cooked (g)	Exact Uncooked (g)
beef	1 oz.	26	34
beef, ground, 80% lean	1.5 oz.	27	41
calamari	1.5 oz.	39	45
Canadian bacon	1 oz.	25	35
catfish	1.5 oz.	38	46
cheese, cheddar	1 oz.	—	29
cheese, cottage	0.25 c.	—	63
cheese, feta	1.5 oz.	—	49
cheese, ricotta	2 oz.	—	62
chicken, breast	1 oz.	23	33
clams	1.5 oz.	27	48
crabmeat	1.5 oz.	39	39
duck	1.5 oz.	30	38
egg substitute, liquid	0.25 c.	—	70
egg, white	2 large	64	64
egg, whole	1 large	52	56
flounder/sole	1.5 oz.	46	56
ham	1 oz.	37	34
lamb, loin	1 oz.	24	34
lamb, ground	1.5 oz.	28	42
lobster	1.5 oz.	37	42
pork, loin chop	1 oz.	27	33
pork, ground	1.5 oz.	27	41
pork, bacon	1 oz.	20	56
salmon	1.5 oz.	28	34
sardines	1 oz.	28	—
scallops	1.5 oz.	34	58
shrimp	1.5 oz.	29	51
soy burgers	0.5 patty	45	—
soy cheese	1 oz.	56	—
soy sausage, links	2 links	37	—
swordfish	1.5 oz.	30	36
tofu, firm	2 oz.	86	—
tofu, soft	3 oz.	107	—
tuna steak	1.5 oz.	24	29
tuna, canned in water	1 oz.	36	—
turkey, breast	1 oz.	23	30
turkey, ground	1.5 oz.	26	36
turkey, deli meat	1.5 oz.	32	—

FATS		
Food	Eyeball	Exact Cooked (g)
NUTS AND SEEDS		
almonds	~ 3	3
almond butter	0.3 tsp.	3
cashews	~ 3	3
macadamia nuts	~ 1	2
peanut butter	0.5 tsp.	3
peanuts	~ 6	3
sunflower seeds	0.25 tsp.	3
walnuts	1 tsp.	2
OTHER		
almond milk, unsweetened	0.5 c.	0.5 c.
avocado	1 tbsp.	10
butter	0.3 tsp.	2
coconut milk	0.5 tbsp.	7
coconut oil	0.3 tsp.	2
cream cheese	1 tsp.	5
cream, heavy	0.3 tsp.	4
cream, light	0.5 tsp.	8
half and half	1 tbsp.	13
lard	0.3 tsp.	2
mayo, light	1 tsp.	5
mayonnaise	0.3 tsp.	2
olive oil	0.3 tsp.	2
olives	~ 5	14
sour cream	1 tsp.	8
tahini	0.3 tsp.	3
tartar sauce	0.5 tsp.	9

Notes:

1) The amount for each item that is required to obtain 7 g of protein, 9 g of carbohydrate, or 1.5 g of fat.

2) Exact data rounded to nearest whole gram.

3) Exact data from USDA Food Composition Databases unless not available therein.

4) Fiber in carbohydrate sources is subtracted to determine a block.

5) * indicates virtually unlimited amounts (over 5 c. for a block).

VEGETABLES

Food	Eyeball	Exact Cooked (g)	Exact Uncooked (g)
acorn squash	0.4 c.	89	100
artichoke	1 small	270	177
arugula	*	—	439
asparagus	12 spears	425	500
bean sprouts	3 c.	265	217
beet green	1.25 c.	351	1450
beets	0.5 c.	112	135
black beans	0.25 c.	60	19
bok choy	3 c.	1,155	761
broccoli	1.25 c.	232	223
Brussels sprouts	0.75 c.	200	174
butternut squash	0.3 c.	123	93
cabbage	1.3 c.	250	272
carrots	0.5 c.	173	132
cauliflower	1.25 c.	500	304
celery	2 c.	375	657
chickpeas	0.25 c.	45	18
collard greens	1.25 c.	545	635
corn	0.25 c.	48	54
cucumber	1 (9 in.)	—	285
dill pickles	3 (3 in.)	—	639
eggplant	1.5 c.	144	313
fava beans	0.3 c.	63	27
green beans	1 c.	193	211
kale	1.25 c.	247	175
kidney beans	0.25 c.	55	26
leeks	1 c.	137	73
lentils	0.25 c.	74	17
lettuce, iceberg	1 head	—	508
lettuce, romaine	6 c.	—	760
lima beans	0.25 c.	65	21
mushrooms	3 c.	291	399
Napa cabbage	5 c.	405	300
okra	0.75 c.	448	212
onion	0.5 c.	103	118
parsnips	0.3 (9 in.)	67	68
peas	0.3 c.	250	180

VEGETABLES

Food	Eyeball	Exact Cooked (g)	Exact Uncooked (g)
peppers, red	1.25 c.	165	230
pinto beans	0.25 c.	52	19
potato, white	0.3 c.	48	68
radicchio	5 c.	—	250
radishes	2 c.	493	500
salsa	0.5 c.	—	190
sauerkraut	1 c.	650	—
snow peas	0.75 c.	211	182
spaghetti squash	1 c.	178	167
spinach	1.3 c.	667	628
summer squash, all	3 c.	309	400
sweet potato	0.3 (5 in.)	52	53
Swiss chard	1.25 c.	443	423
tomato	1 c.	273	335
tomato sauce	0.5 c.	235	—
turnip	0.75 c.	295	195
watercress	*	—	1,140
zucchini	3 c.	536	428

Notes:

1) The amount for each item that is required to obtain 7 g of protein, 9 g of carbohydrate, or 1.5 g of fat.

2) Exact data rounded to nearest whole gram.

3) Exact data from USDA Food Composition Databases unless not available therein.

4) Fiber in carbohydrate sources is subtracted to determine a block.

5) * indicates virtually unlimited amounts (over 5 c. for a block).

FRUITS		
Food	Eyeball	Exact Uncooked (g)
apple	0.5	79
applesauce, unsweetened	0.4 c.	89
apricots	3 small	99
banana	0.3 (9 in.)	45
blackberries	0.5 c.	210
blueberries	0.5 c.	75
cantaloupe	0.25	125
cherries	7	65
cranberries, raw	0.25 c.	117
dates	1	13
figs	0.75	55
grapefruit	0.5	140
grapes	0.5 c.	53
guava	0.5 c.	100
honeydew	0.5	110
kiwi	1	75
kumquat	3	96
mango	0.3 c.	67
nectarine	0.5	102
orange	0.5	99
papaya	0.6 c.	99
peach	1	112
pear	0.5	75
pineapple	0.5 c.	77
plum	1	89
raisins	1 tbsp.	12
raspberries	0.6 c.	167
strawberries	1 c.	160
tangerine	1	78
watermelon	0.5 c.	125

PROCESSED CARBOHYDRATES		
Food	Eyeball	Exact Cooked (g)
bagel	0.25	17
biscuit	0.25	19
bread	0.5 slice	20
bread crumbs	0.5 oz.	20
cereal	0.5 oz.	14
chocolate bar	0.5 oz.	15
cornbread	1-in. square	14
cornstarch	4 tsp.	10
croissant	0.25	21
crouton	0.5 oz.	13
doughnut	0.25	20
English muffin	0.25	21
flour	1.5 tsp.	12
french fries	5	37
graham crackers	1.5	12
granola	0.5 oz.	20
grits	0.3 c.	63
ice cream	0.25 c.	39
melba toast	0.5 oz.	13
oatmeal	0.3 c.	90
pancake	0.5 (4 in.)	32
pasta, cooked	0.25 c.	38
pita bread	0.25	17
popcorn	2 c.	19
potato chips	0.5 c.	18
pretzels	0.5 oz.	12
refried beans	0.25 c.	90
rice	3 tbsp.	32
rice cake	1	12
roll (dinner)	0.5	18
roll (hamburger, hot dog)	0.25	18
saltine crackers	4	13
taco shell	1	16
tortilla (corn)	1 (6 in.)	23
tortilla (flour)	0.5 (6 in.)	20
tortilla chips	0.5 oz.	15
waffle	0.5	27

Notes:

1) The amount for each item that is required to obtain 7 g of protein, 9 g of carbohydrate, or 1.5 g of fat.

2) Exact data rounded to nearest whole gram.

3) Exact data from USDA Food Composition Databases unless not available therein.

4) Fiber in carbohydrate sources is subtracted to determine a block.

5) * indicates virtually unlimited amounts (over 5 c. for a block).

TABLE 4. SAMPLE ZONE MEALS AND SNACKS		
2-BLOCK MENUS		
Breakfast	**Lunch**	**Dinner**
Breakfast Quesadilla 1 corn tortilla 0.25 c. black beans 1 egg (scrambled or fried) 1 oz. cheese 2 tbsp. avocado **Breakfast Sandwich** 0.5 pita bread 1 egg (scrambled or fried) 1 oz. cheese *Served with* 2 macadamia nuts **Fruit Salad** 0.5 c. cottage cheese mixed with 0.25 cantaloupe, cubed 0.5 c. strawberries 0.25 c. grapes *Sprinkled with* 6 chopped almonds **Smoothie** *Blend together:* 1 c. milk 1 tbsp. protein powder 1 c. frozen strawberries 6 cashews **Oatmeal** 0.3 c. cooked oatmeal (slightly watery) 0.5 c. grapes 0.25 c. cottage cheese 2 tsp. walnuts, chopped 1 tbsp. protein powder *Spice with* vanilla extract and cinnamon **Easy Breakfast** 0.5 cantaloupe, cubed 0.5 c. cottage cheese 6 almonds **Steak and Eggs** 1 oz. steak, grilled 1 fried egg 1 slice toast with 0.6 tsp. butter	**Tuna Sandwich** 2 oz. canned tuna 2 tsp. light mayo 1 slice bread **Tacos** 1 corn tortilla 3 oz. seasoned ground meat 0.5 c. tomato, cubed 0.3 c. onion (raw), chopped Lettuce (as garnish), chopped 10 olives, chopped **Deli Sandwich** 1 slice bread 3 oz. sliced deli meat 2 tbsp. avocado **Quesadilla** 1 corn tortilla 2 oz. cheese 2 tbsp. guacamole Jalapeños and salsa as garnish *Serve with* .5 orange **Grilled Chicken Salad** 2 oz. chicken, grilled 2 c. lettuce 0.25 c. tomato, chopped 0.25 cucumber, chopped 0.25 c. green pepper (raw), chopped 0.25 c. black beans 2 tbsp. avocado **Easy Lunch** 3 oz. deli meat 1 apple 2 macadamia nuts	**Fresh Fish** 3 oz. fresh fish, grilled 1.3 c. zucchini (cooked), with herbs *Serve with* large salad with 1 tbsp. salad dressing of choice **Beef Stew** *Sauté:* 0.6 tsp. olive oil 0.3 c. onion (raw), chopped 0.63 c. green pepper (raw), chopped ~4 oz. beef (raw), cubed *Add:* 1.5 c. mushrooms (raw), chopped 0.25 c. tomato sauce *Seasoned with* garlic, Worcestershire sauce, salt and pepper **Chili (serves 3)** *Sauté:* 0.3 c. onion (raw), chopped 0.63 c. green pepper (raw), chopped in garlic, cumin, chili powder, and crushed red peppers *Add:* 9 oz. ground beef, browned 1 c. tomato sauce 0.5 c. black beans 0.25 c. kidney beans 30 olives, chopped *Add* fresh cilantro to taste **Turkey and Greens** 2 oz. turkey breast, roasted 1.25 c. kale, chopped and steamed *Sauté* garlic and crushed red peppers in .66 tsp. olive oil, add the steamed kale and mix. *Serve with* 1 peach, sliced **Easy Chicken Dinner** 2 oz. chicken breast, baked 1 orange 2 macadamia nuts

2-BLOCK MENUS

3-BLOCK MENUS		
Breakfast	**Lunch**	**Dinner**

Breakfast Quesadilla
1 corn tortilla
0.25 c. black beans
0.3 c. onions (raw), chopped
0.63 c. green pepper (raw), chopped
2 eggs (scrambled or fried)
1 oz. cheese
3 tbsp. avocado

Breakfast Sandwich
0.5 pita bread
1 egg (scrambled or fried)
1 oz. cheese
1 oz. sliced ham
Serve with .5 apple and 3 macadamia nuts

Fruit Salad
0.75 c. cottage cheese
0.25 cantaloupe, cubed
1 c. strawberries
0.5 c. grapes
Sprinkle with 9 chopped almonds

Smoothie
Blend together:
1 c. milk
2 tbsp. protein powder
1 c. frozen strawberries
0.5 c. frozen blueberries
9 cashews

Oatmeal
0.6 c. cooked oatmeal (slightly watery)
0.5 c. grapes
0.5 c. cottage cheese
3 tsp. walnuts, chopped
1 tbsp. protein powder
Spice with vanilla extract and cinnamon

Easy Breakfast
0.75 cantaloupe, cubed
0.75 c. cottage cheese
9 almonds

Steak and Eggs
2 oz. steak, grilled
1 fried egg
1 slice toast w/ 1 tsp. butter
0.25 cantaloupe, cubed

Tuna Sandwich
3 oz. canned tuna
3 tsp. light mayo
1 slice bread
Serve with .5 apple

Tacos
2 corn tortillas
3 oz. seasoned ground meat
1 oz. grated cheese
0.5 c. tomato, cubed
0.6 c. onion (raw), chopped
Lettuce (as garnish), chopped
15 olives, chopped

Deli Sandwich
1 slice bread
3 oz. sliced deli meat
1 oz. cheese
3 tbsp. avocado
Serve with .5 apple

Quesadilla
1 corn tortilla
3 oz. cheese
3 tbsp. guacamole
Jalapeños and salsa as garnish
Serve with 1 orange

Grilled Chicken Salad
3 oz. chicken, grilled
2 c. lettuce
0.25 c. tomato, chopped
0.25 cucumber, chopped
0.25 c. green pepper (raw), chopped
0.25 c. black beans
0.25 c. kidney beans
3 tbsp. avocado

Easy Lunch
3 oz. deli meat
1 oz. sliced cheese
1.5 apples
3 macadamia nuts

Fresh Fish
4.5 oz. fresh fish, grilled
1.3 c. zucchini (cooked), with herbs
Serve with large salad with 1.5 tbsp. salad dressing of choice
1 c. strawberries

Beef Stew
Sauté:
1 tsp. olive oil
0.3 c. onion (raw), chopped
0.63 c. green pepper (raw), chopped
~6 oz. beef (raw), cubed
Add:
1.5 c. zucchini (raw), chopped
1.5 c. mushrooms (raw), chopped
0.5 c. tomato sauce
Season with garlic, Worcestershire sauce, salt and pepper

Chili (serves 3)
Sauté:
0.6 c. onion (raw), chopped
1.25 c. green pepper (raw), chopped
in garlic, cumin, chili powder, and crushed red peppers
Add:
13.5 oz. ground beef, browned
1 c. tomato sauce
0.75 c. black beans
0.5 c. kidney beans
45 olives, chopped
Add fresh cilantro to taste

Turkey and Greens
3 oz. turkey breast, roasted
2.5 c. kale, chopped and steamed
Sauté garlic and crushed red peppers in 1 tsp. olive oil, add the steamed kale and mix.
Serve with 1 peach, sliced

Easy Dinner
3 oz. chicken breast, baked
1.5 oranges
3 macadamia nuts

4-BLOCK MENUS		
Breakfast	**Lunch**	**Dinner**

Breakfast	Lunch	Dinner
Breakfast Quesadilla 1 corn tortilla 0.5 c. black beans 0.3 c. onions (raw), chopped 0.63 c. green pepper (raw), chopped 2 eggs (scrambled or fried) 2 oz. cheese 4 tbsp. avocado **Breakfast Sandwich** 0.5 pita bread 2 eggs (scrambled or fried) 1 oz. cheese 1 oz. sliced ham *Serve with* 1 apple and 4 macadamia nuts **Fruit Salad** 1 c. cottage cheese 0.5 cantaloupe, cubed 1 c. strawberries 0.5 c. grapes *Sprinkled with* 12 chopped almonds **Smoothie** *Blend together:* 2 c. milk 2 tbsp. protein powder 1 c. frozen strawberries 0.5 c. frozen blueberries 12 cashews **Oatmeal** 1 c. cooked oatmeal (slightly watery) 0.5 c. grapes 0.75 c. cottage cheese 4 tsp. walnuts, chopped 1 tbsp. protein powder *Spice with* vanilla extract and cinnamon **Easy Breakfast** 1 cantaloupe, cubed 1 c. cottage cheese 12 almonds **Steak and Eggs** 3 oz. steak, grilled 1 fried egg 1 slice bread with 1.3 tsp. butter 0.5 cantaloupe, cubed	**Tuna Sandwich** 4 oz. canned tuna 4 tsp. light mayo 1 slice bread *Serve with* 1 apple **Tacos** 2 corn tortillas 4.5 oz. seasoned ground meat 1 oz. cheese, grated 0.5 c. tomato, cubed 0.3 c. onion (raw), chopped Lettuce (as garnish), chopped 20 olives, chopped *Serve with* .5 apple **Deli Sandwich** 2 slices of bread 4.5 oz. sliced deli meat 1 oz. cheese 4 tbsp. avocado **Quesadilla** 2 corn tortillas 4 oz. cheese 4 tbsp. guacamole Jalapeños and salsa as garnish *Serve with* 1 orange **Grilled Chicken Salad** 4 oz. chicken, grilled 2 c. lettuce 0.25 c. tomato, chopped 0.25 cucumber, chopped 0.25 c. green pepper (raw), chopped 0.5 c. black beans 0.25 c. kidney beans 4 tbsp. avocado **Easy Lunch** 4.5 oz. deli meat 1 oz. cheese 1 apple 1 grapefruit 4 macadamia nuts	**Fresh Fish** 6 oz. fresh fish, grilled 1.3 c. zucchini (cooked), with herbs *Serve with* large salad with 2 tbsp. salad dressing of choice 2 c. strawberries **Beef Stew** *Sauté:* 1.3 tsp. olive oil 0.3 c. onion (raw), chopped 0.63 c. green pepper (raw), chopped ~8 oz. (beef (raw), cubed *Add:* 1.5 c. zucchini (raw), chopped 1.5 c. mushrooms (raw), chopped 1 c. tomato sauce *Season with* garlic, Worcestershire sauce, salt and pepper *Serve with* 1 c. strawberries **Chili (serves 3)** *Sauté:* 0.6 c. onion (raw), chopped 1.25 c. green pepper (raw), chopped in garlic, cumin, chili powder, and crushed red peppers *Add:* 18 oz. ground beef, browned 2 c. tomato sauce 0.75 c. black beans 0.75 c. kidney beans 60 olives, chopped *Add* fresh cilantro to taste **Turkey and Greens** 4 oz. turkey breast, roasted 2.5 c. kale, chopped and steamed *Sauté* garlic and crushed red peppers in 1.3 tsp. olive oil, add kale and mix. *Serve with* 2 peaches, sliced **Easy Dinner** 4 oz. chicken breast, baked 2 oranges 4 macadamia nuts

4-BLOCK MENUS

5-BLOCK MENUS		
Breakfast	**Lunch**	**Dinner**

Breakfast Quesadilla
2 corn tortillas
0.5 c. black beans
0.3 c. onions (raw), chopped
0.63 c. green pepper (raw), chopped
3 eggs (scrambled or fried)
2 oz. cheese
5 tbsp. avocado

Breakfast Sandwich
0.5 pita bread
2 eggs (scrambled or fried)
2 oz. cheese
1 oz. ham, sliced
Serve with 1.5 apples and 5 macadamia nuts

Fruit Salad
1.25 c. cottage cheese
0.5 cantaloupe, cubed
1 c. strawberries
1 c. grapes
Sprinkle with 15 chopped almonds

Smoothie
Blend together:
2 c. milk
3 tbsp. protein powder
2 c. frozen strawberries
0.5 c. frozen blueberries
15 cashews

Oatmeal
1 c. cooked oatmeal (slightly watery)
1 c. grapes
1 c. cottage cheese
5 tsp. walnuts, chopped
1 tbsp. protein powder
Spice with vanilla extract and cinnamon

Easy Breakfast
1.25 cantaloupe, cubed
1.25 c. cottage cheese
~ 15 almonds

Steak and Eggs
3 oz. steak, grilled
2 fried eggs
1 slice bread with 1.6 tsp. butter
0.75 cantaloupe, cubed

Tuna Sandwich
5 oz. canned tuna
5 tsp. light mayo
1 slice bread
Serve with 1.5 apples

Tacos
2 corn tortillas
6 oz. seasoned ground meat
1 oz. cheese, grated
0.5 c. tomato, cubed
0.3 c. onion (raw), chopped
Lettuce (as garnish), chopped
25 olives, chopped
Serve with 1 apple

Deli Sandwich
2 slices bread
4.5 oz. deli meat
2 oz. cheese
5 tbsp. avocado
0.5 apple

Quesadilla
2 corn tortillas
5 oz. cheese
5 tbsp. guacamole
Jalapeños and salsa as garnish
Serve with 1.5 oranges

Grilled Chicken Salad
5 oz. chicken, grilled
2 c. lettuce
0.25 c. tomato, chopped
0.25 cucumber, chopped
0.25 c. green pepper (raw), chopped
0.5 c. black beans
0.5 c. kidney beans
5 tbsp. avocado

Easy Lunch
4.5 oz. deli meat
2 oz. cheese
1.5 apples
1 grapefruit
5 macadamia nuts

Fresh Fish
7.5 oz. fresh fish, grilled
1.3 c. zucchini (cooked), with herbs
Serve with large salad with 0.25 c. black beans and 2.5 tbsp. salad dressing of choice
2 c. strawberries

Beef Stew
Sauté:
1.6 tsp. olive oil
0.6 c. onion (raw), chopped
1.25 c. green pepper (raw), chopped
~10 oz. beef (raw), cubed
Add:
1.5 c. zucchini (raw), chopped
1.5 c. mushrooms (raw), chopped
1 c. tomato sauce
Season with garlic, Worcestershire sauce, salt and pepper
Serve with 2 c. strawberries

Chili (serves 3)
Sauté:
0.6 c. onion (raw), chopped
2.5 c. green pepper (raw), chopped
in garlic, cumin, chili powder, and crushed red peppers
Add:
22.5 oz. ground beef, browned
2 c. tomato sauce
1 c. black beans
1 c. kidney beans
75 olives, chopped
Add fresh cilantro to taste

Turkey and Greens
5 oz. turkey breast, roasted
2.5 c. kale, chopped and steamed
Sauté garlic and crushed red peppers in 1.6 tsp. olive oil, add steamed kale and mix.
Serve with 3 peaches, sliced

Easy Dinner
5 oz. chicken breast, baked
2.5 oranges
5 macadamia nuts

1-BLOCK SNACKS		
1 hard-boiled egg 0.5 orange 6 peanuts	0.5 carrot 3 celery stalks 5 olives	0.25 c. cottage cheese 0.5 c. pineapple 6 peanuts
0.5 c. plain yogurt *Sprinkled with* 3 cashews, chopped	3 oz. soft tofu 0.5 apple 0.5 tsp. peanut butter	1 oz. sardines 0.5 nectarine 5 olives
1 oz. cheese 0.5 apple 1 macadamia nut	1 oz. tuna 1 large tossed salad 1 tsp. salad dressing of choice	1.5 oz. feta cheese 1 c. diced tomato 5 olives
1 oz. canned chicken or tuna 1 peach 0.5 tsp. peanut butter	1 hard boiled egg 1 large spinach salad 1 tsp. salad dressing of choice	1.5 oz. salmon 12 asparagus spears 0.3 tsp. olive oil
1.5 oz. deli-style ham or turkey 1 carrot 5 olives	1 oz. grilled turkey breast 0.5 c. blueberries 3 cashews	1.5 oz. shrimp 2 c. broccoli (raw) 6 peanuts
1 oz. mozzarella string cheese 0.5 c. grapes 1 tbsp. avocado	*Blend:* 1 c. water 1 tbsp. protein powder 0.5 c. grapes 0.3 tsp. coconut oil	1 oz. Canadian bacon 1 plum 1 macadamia nut
1 oz. jack cheese 1 tbsp. guacamole 1 c. tomato 1 c. strawberries 0.25 c. cottage cheese 1 macadamia nut	*Blend:* 1 c. water 0.5 oz. spirulina 1 c. frozen strawberries 3 cashews	1.5 oz. deli-style turkey 1 tangerine 1 tbsp. avocado 0.25 c. cottage cheese 1 c. sliced tomato 0.3 tsp. olive oil
1 poached egg 0.5 slice bread 0.5 tsp. peanut butter	1 oz. cheddar cheese melted over 0.5 apple *Sprinkled with* 1 tsp. walnuts, chopped	1.5 oz. scallops 1 sliced cucumber 0.5 tsp. tartar sauce
0.25 c. cottage cheese		1 oz. lamb 0.25 c. chick peas 0.3 tsp. tahini

1-BLOCK SNACKS

TYPICAL CROSSFIT BLOCK PRESCRIPTIONS AND ADJUSTMENTS

To best understand the Zone Diet, CrossFit athletes should read Dr. Barry Sears' book "Enter the Zone." This article gives more information regarding block prescriptions and fat adjustments for CrossFit athletes.

The chart based on sex and body type in the article "Zone Meal Plans"_is perfect for those who want to start the Zone Diet. If the athlete chooses the wrong block size and does not obtain the desired results, the plan can be modified after a few weeks. Errors in block selection might slow progress, but initial errors are offset by the huge value in starting a practice of weighing and measuring intake.

Sears details a more precise method to calculate one's block prescription in "Enter the Zone." It is:

> Zone block prescription = lean body mass (lb.) x activity level (g/lb. of lean body mass) / 7 (g protein/block)

The activity level ranges on a scale of 0-1. For those who work out several days a week and do not have a labor-intensive job, the activity level should be 0.7 (most CrossFit athletes). By dividing 0.7 by 7 g in the equation, this simplifies to a Zone block prescription that is 10 percent of his or her lean mass.

The activity factor should increase if the athlete does CrossFit two or more times a day, trains for another sport in addition to CrossFit, or holds a strenuous daily job (e.g., construction, farming, etc., and potentially coaching, if on one's feet all day). Although CrossFit workouts are relatively intense, they are not long in duration. An individual does not need to increase the activity level value based on intensity alone; activity volume determines activity factor.

SAMPLE CALCULATION OF THE ZONE BLOCK PRESCRIPTION

Suppose an athlete is 185 lb. (84 kg) with 16 percent body fat. He does CrossFit five days per week and works in a typical office environment. A sample calculation of his Zone block prescription follows.

First, lean body mass is calculated (calipers are a convenient, easy-to-use, and reasonably accurate method):

> lean body mass = 185 lb.–(0.16 x 185 lb.) = 185 lb.–29.6 lb. = 155.4 lb.

Because the activity factor is 0.7, the simplified formula is used:

> block prescription = 155.4 lb. x 0.10 = 15.54 or ~15 blocks

This means that the example athlete above would eat 15 blocks per day (Table 1).

TABLE 1. MACRONUTRIENT AND CALORIE COMPOSITION FOR 15 BLOCKS A DAY		
Protein	15 blocks x 7 g	= 105 g (420 calories)
Carbohydrate	15 blocks x 9 g	= 135 g (540 calories)
Fat	15 blocks x 3 g	= 45 g (405 calories)
Total Calories		= 1,365

Note the total calories presented here are underestimated due to hidden calories. Most foods are classified by a single macronutrient, despite the presence of some other macronutrients (e.g., nuts are classified as a fat but have some protein and carbohydrate calories). These less predominant macronutrients for each source are not included in the total calorie calculations.

This athlete could also choose to round up to 16 blocks, particularly if he or she is more likely to have compliance issues. The Zone prescription is a calorie-restrictive diet and can be especially difficult for new adopters. When one's calculation has a decimal value, rounding up to the next whole block might result in slower progress but produce better long-term compliance. Once the athlete has become accustomed to the diet, then the total blocks can be rounded down to 15, particularly if desired body composition has not been achieved.

INCREASING FAT INTAKE

The caloric restriction leans out the athlete while providing enough protein and carbohydrate for typical CrossFit activity levels. However, the athlete can become too lean. The athlete is considered "too lean" when performance decreases in combination with continued weight loss. "Too lean" should not be based on body weight or appearance alone. When a loss of mass coincides with a drop in performance, the athlete needs to add calories to the diet. This can be accomplished by doubling the fat intake (Table 2).

TABLE 2. MACRONUTRIENT AND CALORIE COMPOSITION FOR 15 BLOCKS A DAY AND TWO TIMES FAT		
Protein	15 blocks x 7 g	= 105 g (420 calories)
Carbohydrate	15 blocks x 9 g	= 135 g (540 calories)
Fat	30 blocks x 3 g	= 90 g (810 calories)
Total Calories		= 1,770

At twice the fat, the macronutrient ratio based on calories has changed from 30 percent protein, 40 percent carbohydrate, 30 percent fat to 23 percent protein, 31 percent carbohydrate, 46 percent fat. Fat can continue to be multiplied if the athlete experiences further mass loss and performance decline. Some CrossFit athletes have a diet including five times the fat (Table 3).

TABLE 3. MACRONUTRIENT AND CALORIE COMPOSITION FOR 15 BLOCKS A DAY AND FIVE TIMES FAT		
Protein	15 blocks x 7 g	= 105 g (420 calories)
Carbohydrate	15 blocks x 9 g	= 135 g (540 calories)
Fat	75 blocks x 3 g	= 225 g (2,025 calories)
Total Calories		= 2,985

At five times the fat, the macronutrient ratio based on calories has changed to 14 percent protein, 18 percent carbohydrate, 68 percent fat. ▪

SUPPLEMENTATION

Whole, unprocessed foods are the best source of both macronutrients and micro-nutrients in terms of composition, variety, and density, such that supplementation is generally not recommended. We contend that eating a diet composed of known quantities and of high-quality whole foods is the most important aspect of nutrition for improved performance and health. Not only are supplements generally poorer nutrient sources, but they are also an unnecessary focus for someone not following our basic diet plan of weighed and measured meat and vegetables, etc.

However, we find one supplement beneficial enough to make a blanket recommendation: fish oil. Fish oil provides omega-3 fatty acids, which are a type of poly-unsaturated fat.

Physiological fats are known as triglycerides in biological terms; they are composed of a glycerol backbone with three fatty acids attached (Figure 1). The attached fatty acids are mixtures of saturated, monounsaturated, and polyunsaturated fats. Although one fatty acid is prominent in each food, all three are represented to some degree. Figure 2 provides a summary of the types of fat and example food sources.

The two types of polyunsaturated fats found most frequently in foods are omega-3 and omega-6 fats. Classifying a fatty acid as omega-3 versus omega-6 is dependent on chemical structure. Polyunsaturated fats are sources of the two essential fatty acids, meaning they must be obtained from the diet. They are alpha-linolenic acid (ALA) (an omega-3) and linoleic acid (LA) (an omega-6). Omega-3 fats are known as "anti-inflammatory" fats, and omega-6 fats are known as "pro-inflammatory" fats based on their physiological functions. Both are needed in relatively equal quantities.

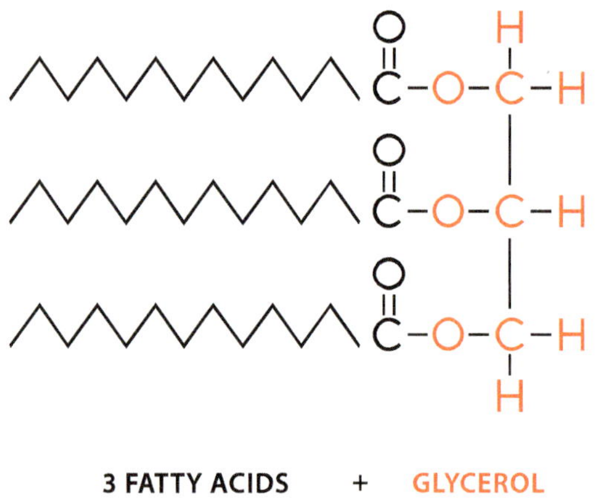

3 FATTY ACIDS   +   GLYCEROL

Figure 1. Fat in Food is in the Form of a Triglyceride.

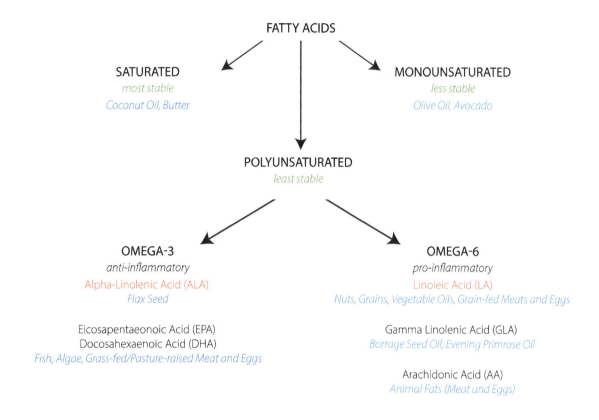

Figure 2. Summary of Fatty Acids and Example Food Sources.

Current diets tend to have too many omega-6 fats, pushing the balance toward pro-inflammatory physiological processes. The current omega-6:omega-3 ratio is approximately 20:1 and higher, where primitive populations likely had a ratio closer to 2:1. Sources of omega-6 fats in the diet are vegetable oils, nuts, conventionally raised (grain-fed/feed-lot) meat and eggs, and farm-raised fish. Eliminating processed food from our diet should reduce exposure to omega-6 fats from vegetable oils. However, most meat and eggs are conventionally raised, which results in greater omega-6 content than if they were wild or grass fed. Nuts and seeds also have more omega-6 fats than omega-3. Therefore, it is possible that even though one eats the foods on our list, his or her diet could still be pro-inflammatory relative to the ancestral past.

Fish-oil supplementation improves the ratio of omega-6 to omega-3 fatty acids and reduces the inflammatory responses in the body. Fish oil provides two types of omega-3 fatty acids: eicosapentaenoic acid (EPA) and docosahexaenoic acid (DHA), the form of omega-3 fats preferred by the brain and body. The body can convert ALA to EPA and DHA, but the conversion process is inefficient. Some practitioners have recommended a combined daily intake on the order of 3 grams of EPA and DHA for an otherwise healthy individual, although the exact amount is dictated by one's total omega-6 intake. Each brand of fish oil has a different concentration of EPA and DHA per serving as indicated on the label. Individuals might have to take multiple servings to get 3 grams of EPA and DHA, as brands might include omega-3s that are neither EPA nor DHA (e.g., ALA). Flax seed or oil is not an appropriate supplement for omega-3s. Flax is a good source of ALA, but because of the poor conversion to EPA and DHA, it is not recommended. If the individual is vegan, DHA can be obtained with algae oil.

Research has indicated positive health benefits by supplementing with fish oil. Omega-3 fats help increase the fluidity of cell membranes, and research has indicated supplementation can improve insulin sensitivity, cardiovascular function, nervous-system function, immune health, memory, and mood issues. Omega 3s also function as an anti-coagulant, so military personnel should consider removing fish oil supplements from their diet a couple of weeks prior to deployment. It might also be appropriate for those with an upcoming surgery to stop taking fish oil two weeks from that date. These individuals should talk with their doctor regarding these circumstances.

It is possible to avoid omega-3 supplementation depending on food intake, although the individual needs to be fastidious with his or her diet. This could be accomplished by avoidance of all vegetable oils (which are used at most every restaurant), and nuts and seeds. Meat would have to be grass-fed and eggs pasture-raised, and wild-caught fish should be consumed a few times a week. Because this is not practical for many people, supplementation is effective.

Besides the ratio of omega-6 to omega-3s in the diet, the total amount of polyunsaturated fat is an important consideration. It is not ideal to take in high doses of either omega-6 (vegetable oils, nuts) or omega-3 fats (based on the stability of polyunsaturated fats relative to other fats, Figure 2). Fish oil supplementation does not negate the effects of a bad diet (e.g., eating fast food or excessive amounts of nuts and nut butters). The total recommended polyunsaturated fat intake in a diet is not well established; an equal representation of the three fats appears prudent. Individuals should work with a primary care doctor to determine if supplementation is appropriate, particularly in cases with specific medical conditions. ▪

A THEORETICAL TEMPLATE FOR CROSSFIT'S PROGRAMMING

Originally published in February 2003.

"What is Fitness? (Part 1)" explores the aims and objectives of our program. Most of you have a clear understanding of how we implement our program through familiarity with the Workout of the Day (WOD) from our website. What is likely less clear is the rationale behind the WOD or more specifically what motivates the specifics of CrossFit's programming. It is our aim in this article to offer a model or template for our workout programming in the hope of elaborating on the CrossFit concept and potentially stimulating productive thought on the subject of exercise prescription (generally) and workout construction (specifically). What we want to do is bridge the gap between an understanding of our philosophy of fitness and the workouts themselves; that is, how we get from theory to practice. CrossFit.com has never used this template for its programming, but it provides new trainers a way to effectively apply variance within the tenets of CrossFit's methodology.

At first glance, the template seems to be offering a routine or regimen. This might seem at odds with our contention that workouts need considerable variance or unpredictability to best mimic the often unforeseeable challenges that combat, sport, and survival demand and reward. We have often said, "What your regimen needs is to not become routine." But the model we offer allows for wide variance of mode, exercise, metabolic pathway, rest, intensity, sets, and reps. In fact, it is mathematically likely that each three-day cycle is a singularly unique stimulus never to be repeated in a lifetime of CrossFit workouts.

The template is engineered to allow for a wide and constantly varied stimulus, randomized within some parameters, but still true to the aims and purposes of CrossFit. Our template contains sufficient structure to formalize or define our programming objectives while not setting in stone parameters that must be left to variance if the workouts are going to meet our needs. That is our mission–to ideally blend structure and flexibility.

It is not our intention to suggest that your workouts should, or that our workouts do, fit neatly and cleanly within the template, for that is absolutely not the case. But, the template does offer sufficient structure to aid comprehension, reflect the bulk of our programming concerns, and not hamstring the need for radically varying stimulus. So as not to seem redundant, what we are saying here is that the purpose of the template is as much descriptive as prescriptive.

TEMPLATE MACRO VIEW

In the broadest view we see a three-days-on, one-day-off pattern. We have found that this allows for a relatively higher volume of high-intensity work than the many others that we have experimented with. With this format the athlete can work at or near the highest intensities possible for three straight days, but by the fourth

The magic is in the movement, the art is in the programming, the science is in the explanation, and the fun is in the community."

–COACH GLASSMAN

TABLE 1. TEMPLATE MACRO VIEW 3-DAYS-ON, 1-DAY-OFF												
Day	1	2	3	4	5	6	7	8	9	10	11	12
Modality	M	G W	M G W	OFF	G	W M	G W M	OFF	W	M G	W M G	OFF

5-DAYS-ON, 2-DAYS-OFF						
Day	1	2	3	4	5	6	7
Week 1	M	G W	M G W	M G	W	OFF	OFF
Week 2	G	W M	G W M	G W	M	OFF	OFF
Week 3	W	M G	W M G	W M	G	OFF	OFF

Modalities

M = monostructural metabolic conditioning

G = gymnastics

W = weightlifting

day both neuromuscular function and anatomy are hammered to the point where continued work becomes noticeably less effective and impossible without reducing intensity.

The chief drawback to the three-days-on, one-day-off regimen is that it does not sync with the five-days-on, two-days-off pattern that seems to govern most of the world's work habits. The regimen is at odds with the seven-day week. Many of our clients are running programs within professional settings, where the five-day workweek with weekends off is de rigueur. Others have found that the scheduling needs of family, work, and school require scheduling workouts on specific days of the week every week. For these people we have devised a five-days-on, two-days-off regimen that has worked very well.

The workout of the day was originally a five-on, two-off pattern and it worked perfectly. But the three-on, one-off pattern was devised to increase both the intensity of and recovery from the workouts, and the feedback we have received and our observations suggest that it was successful in this regard.

If life is easier with the five-on, two-off pattern, do not hesitate to employ it. The difference in potential between the two might not warrant restructuring your entire life to accommodate the more effective pattern. There are other factors that will ultimately overshadow any disadvantages inherent in the potentially less effective regimen, such as convenience, attitude, exercise selection, and pacing.

For the remainder of this article the three-day cycle is the one in discussion, but most of the analysis and discussion applies perfectly to the five-day cycle.

ELEMENTS BY MODALITY

Looking at the Template Macro View (Table 1) it can readily be seen that the template is based on the rotation of three distinct modalities: monostructural metabolic conditioning (M), gymnastics (G), and weightlifting (W). The monostructural metabolic conditioning activities are commonly referred to as "cardio," the purpose of which is primarily to improve cardiorespiratory capacity and stamina. They are repetitive, cyclical movements that could be sustained for long periods of time. The gymnastics modality comprises body-weight exercises/elements or calisthenics, and its primary purpose is to improve body control by improving neurological components such as coordination, balance, agility, and accuracy, and to improve functional upper-body capacity and trunk strength. The weightlifting modality comprises the most important weight-training basics, Olympic lifts and powerlifting, where the aim is primarily to increase strength, power, and hip/leg capacity. This category includes any exercise with the addition of an external load.

Table 2 gives the common exercises used by our program, separated by modality, in fleshing out the routines.

For metabolic conditioning the exercises are run, bike, row, and jump rope. The gymnastics modality includes air squats, pull-ups, push-ups, dips, handstand push-ups, rope climbs, muscle-ups, presses to handstands, back/hip extensions, sit-ups, and jumps (vertical, box, broad, etc.). The weightlifting modality includes

TABLE 2. EXERCISES BY MODALITY		
Gymnastics	**Metabolic Conditioning**	**Weightlifting**
Air Squat	Run	Deadlift
Pull-up	Bike	Cleans
Push-up	Row	Press
Dip	Jump Rope	Snatch
Handstand Push-up		Clean and Jerk
Rope Climb		Medicine-Ball Drills
Muscle-up		Kettlebell Swing
Press to Handstand		
Back Extension		
Sit-up		
Jump		
Lunge		

deadlifts, cleans, presses, snatches, clean and jerks, medicine-ball drills and throws, and kettlebell swings.

The elements, or exercises, chosen for each modality were selected for their functionality, neuroendocrine response, and overall capacity to dramatically and broadly impact the human body.

WORKOUT STRUCTURE

The workout structure varies by the inclusion of one, two, or three modalities for each day (Table 3). Days 1, 5, and 9 are each single-modality workouts whereas days 2, 6, and 10 include two modalities each (couplets), and finally, days 3, 7, and 11 use three modalities each (triplets). In every case each modality is represented by a single exercise or element; i.e., each M, W, and G represents a single exercise from metabolic conditioning, weightlifting, and gymnastics modalities respectively.

When the workout includes a single exercise (days 1, 5, and 9) the focus is on a single exercise or effort. When the element is the single "M" (day 1) the workout is a single effort and is typically a long, slow, distance effort. When the modality is a single "G" (day 5) the workout is practice of a single skill, and typically this skill is sufficiently complex to require great practice but might not be yet suitable for inclusion in a timed workout because performance is not yet adequate for efficient inclusion. When the modality is the single "W" (day 9) the workout is a single lift and typically performed at high weight and low repetition. It is worth repeating that the focus on days 1, 5, and 9 is single efforts of "cardio" at long distance; improving high-skill, more complex gymnastics movements; and single/low-rep heavy weightlifting basics, respectively. This is not the day to work sprints, pull-ups, or high-repetition clean and jerks—the other days would be more appropriate.

> A strength and conditioning regimen devoid of gymnastics practice and skills is deficient."
>
> –COACH GLASSMAN

TABLE 3. WORKOUT STRUCTURE			
Days	**Single-Element Days (1, 5, 9)**	**Two-Element Days (2, 6, 10)**	**Three-Element Days (3, 7, 11)**
Priority	Element priority	Task priority	Time priority
Structure (Set Structure)	M: Single effort G: Single skill W: Single lift	Couplet repeated 3-5 times for time	Triplet repeated for 20 minutes for rotations
Intensity	M: Long, slow distance G: High skill W: Heavy	Two moderately to intensely challenging elements	Three lightly to moderately challenging elements
Work Recovery Character	Recovery not a limiting factor	Work/rest interval management critical	Work/rest interval marginal factor

Day	Modality	Elements
TABLE 4. WORKOUT EXAMPLES USING THE TEMPLATE		
1	M	Run 10 km
2	G W	(5 handstand push-ups/225 x 5 deadlifts + 20 lb./round) x 5 for time
3	M G W	Run 400 m/10 pull-ups/thruster 50% of body weight (BW) x 15 for 20 min. for rotations
4	OFF	
5	G	Practice handstands for 45 minutes
6	W M	(Bench press 75% BW x 10/Row 500 m) x 5 for time
7	G W M	Lunges 100 ft./push press 50% BW x 15/row 500 m for 20 min. for rotations
8	OFF	
9	W	Deadlift 5-3-3-2-2-2-1-1-1
10	M G	(Run 200 m/box jump 30 in. x 10) x 5 for time
11	W M G	Clean 50% BW x 20/bike 1 mile/15 push-ups for 20 min. for rotations
12	OFF	

On the single-element days (1, 5, and 9), recovery is not a limiting factor. For the "G" and "W" days, rest is long and deliberate and the focus is kept clearly on improvement of the element and not on total metabolic effect.

For the two-element days (2, 6, and 10), the structure is typically a couplet of exercises performed alternately until repeated for a total of 3-5 rounds performed for time. We say these days are "task priority" because the task is set and the time varies. The workout is most often scored by the time required to complete the prescribed rounds. The two elements themselves are designed to be moderate to high intensity and work-rest interval management is critical. These elements are made intense by pace, load, reps or some combination. Ideally, the first round is hard but possible, whereas the second and subsequent rounds will require pacing, rest, and breaking the task up into manageable efforts.

For the three-element days (3, 7, and 11), the structure is typically a triplet of exercises, this time repeated for a specified number of minutes and scored by number of rotations or repetitions completed. We say these workouts are "time priority" because the athlete is kept moving for a specified time and the goal is to complete as many cycles as possible. The elements are chosen in order to provide a challenge that manifests only through repeated cycles. Ideally the elements chosen

No successful strength and conditioning program has anywhere ever been derived from scientific principles. Those claiming efficacy or legitimacy on the basis of theories they've either invented or corralled to explain their programming are guilty of fraud. Programming derives from clinical practice and can only be justified or legitimized by the results of that practice."

–COACH GLASSMAN

are not significant outside of the blistering pace required to maximize rotations completed within the time allotted (typically 20 minutes). This is in stark contrast to the two-element days, where the elements are of a much higher intensity. This workout is tough, extremely tough, but managing work-rest intervals is a marginal factor.

Each of the three distinct days has a distinct character. Generally speaking, as the number of elements increases from one to two to three, the workout's effect is due less to the individual element selected and more to the effect of repeated efforts. Table 4 depicts workout examples following this template.

APPLICATION

The template in discussion does not generate the CrossFit.com Workout of the Day (WOD), but the qualities of one-, two-, and three-element workouts expressed there motivated the template's design. Our experience in the gym and the feedback from our athletes following the WOD have demonstrated that the mix of one-, two-, and three-element workouts is crushing in impact and unrivaled in bodily response. The information garnered through your feedback on the WOD has given CrossFit an advantage in estimating and evaluating the effect of workouts that might have taken decades or been impossible without the internet.

Typically our most effective workouts, like art, are remarkable in composition, symmetry, balance, theme, and character. There is a "choreography" of exertion that draws from a working knowledge of physiological response, a well-developed sense of the limits of human performance, the use of effective elements, experimentation, and even luck. Our hope is that this model will aid in learning this art.

The template encourages new skill development, generates unique stressors, crosses modes, incorporates quality movements, and hits all three metabolic pathways. It does this within a framework of sets and reps and a cast of exercises that CrossFit has repeatedly tested and proven effective. We contend that this template does a reasonable job of formally expressing many CrossFit objectives and values. ▪

SCALING CROSSFIT

CrossFit workouts, and especially those on CrossFit.com, are designed to challenge even the most advanced athlete. Many athletes need to "scale" (i.e., modify) the workouts for the safest implementation of the program. Finding a CrossFit affiliate is one way to receive proper coaching and guidance through this process. In absence of an experienced trainer, this article presents some basic concepts for scaling workouts particularly for beginners. Scaling for other populations (e.g., advanced or injured athletes) is discussed in greater detail at the Level 2 Certificate Course, as well as in the Online Scaling Course.

Athletes will need to scale workouts for variable lengths of time. One's athletic background, as well as his or her current health and fitness capacity, dictates how long scaling is necessary. The methodology presented here can be used indefinitely, but a month is the minimum period for which significant scaling should be applied. This introductory period serves two purposes: 1) it develops competency of movements used in CrossFit; and 2) it appropriately exposes the athlete to gradual increases in intensity and volume.

MECHANICS AND CONSISTENCY FIRST

CrossFit's charter for creating the most optimal balance of safety, efficacy, and efficiency is: mechanics, consistency, then—and only then—intensity. The initial exposure to CrossFit is when movement mechanics should be prioritized over intensity. And for some, just practicing the movements will be intense. It is imperative that the movements can be performed correctly and consistently before load and speed are added. While intensity is an important part of the CrossFit program, it is added after movement proficiency is established. Ignoring this order increases the risk for injury and potentially blunts long-term progress, especially if poor mechanics are combined with load.

SCALING EFFECTIVELY: PRESERVE THE STIMULUS

When scaling workouts, the main principle to follow is "preserve the stimulus." The stimulus of the workout refers to the effects of the specific combination of movements, time domain, and load. Aspects of this combination can be adjusted for each individual so that the workout produces relatively similar effects on each athlete—regardless of physical abilities.

The breadth of workouts and varying levels of CrossFit beginners make it impossible to provide a single rule for scaling workouts. Similarly, deviations from the guidelines presented herein can be effective choices at times (especially for more advanced athletes). For best results, the individual should use his or her own judgment—or the advice of a qualified trainer—to determine what is appropriate. Athletes and trainers should not be afraid to alter the workout after it has begun. At the appearance of unsafe form, the athlete or coach should end the workout or reduce the load to that which allows proper mechanics.

Intensity and Volume

Two factors need to be scaled for every beginner: 1) intensity; and 2) volume. A prudent method for beginners is reducing intensity and/or volume by half for at least two weeks. Depending on how the athlete progresses, volume and intensity can be gradually increased in the following weeks, months, and years.

Intensity refers to the amount of power an athlete generates. Intensity may be modified in three ways: 1) load; 2) speed; and/or 3) volume.

Load is the variable to scale first; scaling the load is an easy way to preserve the stimulus relative to an athlete's capacity. Load is also the most common variable modified after the beginner period. Especially for a conditioning workout, the athlete should use a load that ensures he or she is able to complete the first set or round without compromising form or reaching muscular failure. Determining appropriate loads for newer athletes requires some estimation, and scaling will not always be perfect. Often, loads for newer athletes will be less than 50 percent of the prescribed load, especially if an athlete is new to lifting weights. Coaches should err on the side of scaling too much rather than not enough, particularly for newer athletes.

Speed tends to be more self-modulated due to the athlete's fitness level, although a coach can modulate speed based on the mechanics demonstrated. A coach might have to slow an athlete down to achieve the correct mechanics. Similarly, coaches might have to encourage an athlete who is moving well to move faster, though this is less common when working with beginners (see "Technique" article).

Volume is the total amount of work accomplished by the athlete. Depending on the workout, volume can be lowered by reducing: 1) time; 2) reps/rounds; and/or 3) distance.

Newer CrossFit athletes might attempt to struggle through a workout where the volume of repetitions (or load, above) is beyond their current capacity. For example, an advanced CrossFit athlete might complete Fran in 2 minutes. That same workout might take a newer athlete 15 minutes or more if completed as prescribed. While it is not imperative for beginners to finish in the same time as advanced athletes – times should be relatively similar. Fran should be completed within several minutes.

While lowering the volume can increase intensity (i.e., produce more power), volume reductions are also important for beginners because muscles, ligaments, and tendons need to become gradually accustomed to the volume in CrossFit. Reducing volume also reduces excessive soreness, as well as the risk for rhabdomyolysis and injury.

Movements

When a movement cannot be performed at all, it can be substituted. CrossFit suggests modifying this variable last because avoiding a movement prevents an individual from developing proficiency in it. An athlete or trainer should first try reducing the load before substituting the movement. If the workout calls for snatches at 95 lb., for example, it is generally preferable that the athlete performs the snatches with a PVC pipe instead of substituting 95-lb. overhead squats.

Complete movement substitutions should be considered when a physical limitation or injury is present, or when the load cannot be reduced. When selecting a substitute movement, trainers should try to preserve the original movement's function and range of motion as best they can. When determining movement substitutions consider:

1) Whether the movement is primarily driven by the lower body or upper body.
2) The movement function (e.g., push versus pull).
3) The range of motion used by the movement (specifically of the hips, knees, and ankles).
4) The plane of movement.

Particularly in the case of injury, a complete movement replacement might be necessary. Consideration of these variables can help trainers select a movement substitution or replacement that is as similar as possible to the prescribed movement.

A SAMPLE WEEK OF SCALING

This section outlines five typical CrossFit workouts. For each Workout of the Day (WOD), scaled workouts are presented with modifications to volume, load, and movements. Some of the rationale for the options is also described. These scaled workouts should be considered but three examples of the many options available. They do not take the place of scaled workouts created by an experienced trainer who is relying on intuition and detailed knowledge of a specific athlete.

WORKOUT 1

CINDY	SCALED VERSION A	SCALED VERSION B	SCALED VERSION C
As many rounds as possible (AMRAP) in 20 minutes of: 5 pull-ups 10 push-ups 15 air squats	*10-minute AMRAP of:* 5 ring rows 10 push-ups from knees 15 air squats to a target	*10-minute AMRAP of:* 5 jumping pull-ups 10 push-ups against a wall 15 air squats	*10 rounds for time of:* 3 pull-ups with bands 6 push-ups from toes 9 air squats

Scaling Considerations

- Volume is reduced by halving the time or setting an upper limit of rounds.
- The rep range can also be reduced so the individual keeps moving through most of the workout instead of reaching muscular failure too quickly.
- Pull-ups and push-ups often exceed the upper-body strength of beginning athletes, and these movements can be scaled in various ways to reduce the load.
- Air squats should be maintained unless there is an injury, although a target is useful for those developing full range of motion.

WORKOUT 2

	SCALED VERSION A	SCALED VERSION B	SCALED VERSION C
50-40-30-20-10 reps for time of: Wall-ball shots, 20-lb. ball Box jumps, 24-in. box	*25-20-15-10-5 reps for time of:* Wall-ball shots, 20-lb. ball Box jumps, 24-in. box	*50-40-30-20-10 reps for time of:* Wall-ball shots, 14-lb. ball *25-20-15-10-5 reps for time of:* Box jumps, 24-in. box	*5 rounds for time of:* *15 Wall-ball shots, 10-lb. ball* 15 Plate jumps, 45-lb. plate

Scaling Considerations

- The total volume of this workout is relatively high for each movement (150 reps). Controlling the reps is the easiest way to reduce the volume.
- It is also possible to reduce volume on one movement only. For example, if the athlete is attempting box jumps at a certain height for the first time this can be reduced while keeping the wall-ball shots at the prescribed volume.
- The box height can be significantly reduced to help preserve the jump. Step-ups could be used to preserve the range of motion when capacity does allow for jumps (e.g., injury).
- Also consider changing the height to which the wall ball is thrown, particularly when the athlete is new to the movement and/or trying a new weight.

WORKOUT 3

DEADLIFT	SCALED VERSION A	SCALED VERSION B	SCALED VERSION C
5-5-5-5-5	*Everyone works up to heavy set of 5 repetitions with sound mechanics. The set should be taxing, but form should not be lost.*		

Scaling Considerations

- When the heavy day has a low repetition count per set (<5 reps), trainers might choose to increase the repetitions for beginners who are working at a lower weight to practice mechanics. For example, a 1-repetition-maximum snatch day may be changed to 3 repetitions.
- In rare cases, the range of motion may be shortened until the mechanics are correct. This might require the barbell to be pulled from pins (or off bumpers), for example. Typically, however, beginners should work on improving mechanics through the full range of motion.

WORKOUT 4

	SCALED VERSION A	SCALED VERSION B	SCALED VERSION C
21-18-15-12-9-6-3 reps of: Sumo deadlift high pulls (SDHP) (75 lb.) Push jerks (75 lb.)	*15-12-9-6-3 reps of:* SDHP (45 lb.) Push jerks (45 lb.)	*15-12-9-6-3 reps of:* SDHP (1-pood/36-lb. kettlebell) Push presses (45 lb.)	*5 rounds for time of:* 10 SDHP (45 lb.) 10 Push jerks (45 lb.)

Scaling Considerations

The total volume is moderately high (84 reps) and is effectively halved by removing the first two rounds of 21 and 18 reps.

- The load can be reduced for both movements. As they are more complicated movements for beginners, this is a perfect opportunity to keep the movements as is but lower the load to refine the mechanics.
- In rare cases, a push press should be substituted when the mechanics of the push jerk are not proficient for significant load or volume.
- Substituting a kettlebell for a barbell in the SDHP is a way to reduce the complexity of the movement. It allows the athletes to work on the core-to-extremity movement pattern without having to navigate a bar around the knees.

WORKOUT 5

	SCALED VERSION A	SCALED VERSION B	SCALED VERSION C
12-9-6 reps of: Cleans (185 lb.) Muscle-ups	*12-9-6 reps of:* Cleans (75 lb.) Banded strict pull-ups Banded strict dips	*12-9-6 reps of:* Medicine-ball cleans (20 lb.) Ring rows Bench dips	*3 rounds for time of:* 8 cleans (95 lb.) 8 banded muscle-up transitions

Scaling Considerations

- The total volume of this workout is low without any modifications.
- The load is significantly heavy and will need to be reduced for beginners. A medicine ball is particularly useful for the newer athlete.
- The muscle-up will need to be scaled, and this is best accomplished with upper-body pulling and pushing movements, or even a banded version of the full movement itself.
- Changing the rep scheme can be useful when the modification significantly challenges the individual's strength stamina. Doing so will allow the individual to achieve almost the same volume while he or she develops new skills and/or is exposed to heavier elements.

CONCLUSION

Athletes and their trainers should focus on movement proficiency before adding speed and load. Workouts should be scaled significantly for at least a month, particularly with regard to intensity and volume. The period of scaling workouts—especially load—might continue for months and years as the athlete develops the requisite capacities. With appropriate scaling, an athlete will make significant fitness gains by working at his or her relative level of physical and psychological tolerance.

Most athletes need to modify CrossFit.com workouts to dose themselves appropriately. As mentioned in "Where Do I Go From Here?" we challenge all athletes and trainers to follow CrossFit.com for their daily workouts for at least six months. Following this recommendation will provide first-hand experience at scaling workouts. ▪

"THE GIRLS" FOR GRANDMAS

Originally published in October 2004.

As a demonstration of the program's universal applicability, this article gives scaled variations of benchmark workouts Angie, Barbara, Chelsea, Diane, Elizabeth, and Fran.

These six workouts are as good as any to demonstrate our concept of scalability. Here we offer versions of those workouts that have been "tuned down" in intensity and had exercises substituted to accommodate any audience, particularly the elderly, beginner, or deconditioned athlete.

With scaling, the intent is to preserve the stimulus: adhere to as many of the original workout factors as possible relative to the individual's physical and psychological tolerances.

ANGIE	
ORIGINAL	**SCALED**
For time:	*For time:*
100 pull-ups	25 ring rows
100 push-ups	25 push-ups off the knees
100 sit-ups	25 sit-ups
100 squats	25 squats

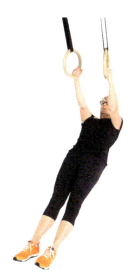 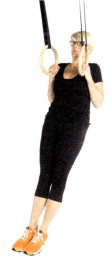

Ring Rows

BARBARA

ORIGINAL	SCALED
5 rounds for time of:	*3 rounds for time of:*
20 pull-ups	20 ring rows
30 push-ups	30 push-ups off the knees
40 sit-ups	40 sit-ups
50 squats	50 squats
3 minutes of rest between rounds	*3 minutes of rest between rounds*

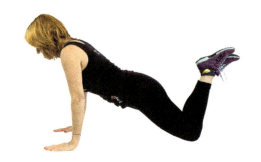
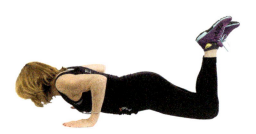

Push-ups off the Knees

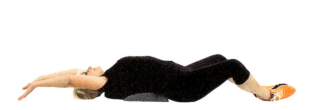
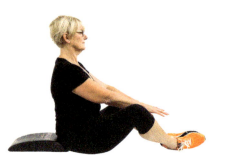

Sit-ups

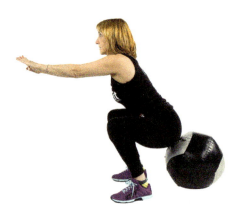

Squats

CHELSEA

ORIGINAL	SCALED
5 pull-ups 10 push-ups 15 squats *Each minute on the minute for 30 minutes*	5 ring rows 10 push-ups off the knees 15 squats *Each minute on the minute for 20 minutes*

DIANE

ORIGINAL	SCALED

21-15-9 repetitions (reps) for time of:
    deadlift 225 lb.
    handstand push-ups
	21-15-9 reps for time of:
	    deadlift 50 lb.
	    dumbbell shoulder press 10 lb.

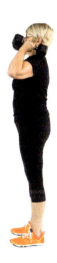 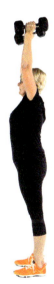

Dumbbell Shoulder Press

FRAN

ORIGINAL	SCALED

21-15-9 reps for time of:
    thruster 95 lb.
    pull-ups
	21-15-9 reps for time of:
	    thruster 25 lb.
	    ring rows

ELIZABETH	
ORIGINAL	**SCALED**

21-15-9 reps for time of:
    clean 135 lb.
    ring dips
	21-15-9 reps for time of:
	    clean 25 lb.
	    bench dips

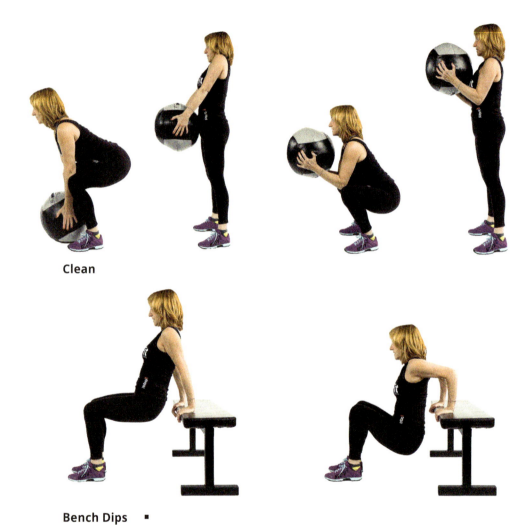

Clean

Bench Dips ▪

RUNNING A CROSSFIT CLASS

At most affiliates, group classes outnumber private or semi-private sessions. This is a short primer on how to effectively plan and run a group class. While the concepts presented here are relevant to private training, the logistical demands of running a group class are significantly increased such that additional pressure is placed on planning.

More information on designing and running effective classes is provided in the Level 2 Certificate Course. Programming well-designed workouts and providing scaling options are only part of running an effective class. At the very least, a warm-up, workout, and cool-down plan should be drafted before the class to outline the duration of each section and its specific elements. Additional considerations for each section are outlined below.

Does the warm-up...
- Increase the body's core temperature?
- Prepare the athletes to handle the intensity of the workout?
- Allow the coach to correct movement mechanics needed in the workout?
- Allow the coach to assess capacity for scaling modifications?
- Offer skill development and refinement (potentially including elements not in the workout, time permitting)?

Does the workout...
- Include a description of range-of-motion standards?
- Include scaling options that are appropriate for all athletes in the class?
- Allow athletes to reach their relative level of high intensity?
- Challenge the athlete's current level of fitness?
- Include corrections of movement mechanics under high intensity?

Does the cool-down...
- Allow the heart and respiratory rate to slow and the athlete to regain mental acuity?
- Allow the athlete to record workout performance to track progress?
- Prepare the gym for the following class?
- Take advantage of remaining time for recovery practices, additional skill refinement, and/or education?

The following three sample Lesson Plans and Workout of the Day (WOD) Scales serve as examples for how to plan a class session. ▪

LESSON PLAN: FRAN

WORKOUT
Fran
21-15-9 reps of:
95-lb. thrusters
Pull-ups

Score: total time

INTENDED STIMULUS
This workout is classic benchmark that allows coaches and athletes to assess progress. Fran, a couplet of gymnastics and weightlifting movements, is a relatively fast workout elite athletes finish in less than 2 minutes.

The complementary movement patterns—lower-body push and upper-body pull—allow for relatively continuous movement. The greatest challenge is managing an extremely high heart rate.

BREAKDOWN

- This workout is more a challenge of one's cardiovascular response than strength. Athletes should not need to break these movements up more than three times in the set of 21, two times in the set of 15, and once in the set of 9.

- The suggested female Rx'd weight is 65 lb. for the thruster.

- The scaling options include: reduced load on the thruster, and/or reduced volume or load on the pull-ups. If an athlete's last Fran was scaled and completed under 5 minutes, difficulty should be increased.

- Coaches should demonstrate each movement including movement standards.

- Coaches should explain the score is total time for workout completion.

- Coaches should ask if any athletes are injured.

- Athletes should attempt to complete the workout in less than 10 minutes. The approximate estimates of each component are: 30-90 seconds for each set of 21, 20-60 seconds for each set of 15, and 15-45 seconds for each set of 9.

Coaches: All parts of the class are coach led. Demonstrate each new piece before athletes perform it. Cue athletes to achieve better positions throughout each section.

:00–:03
WHITEBOARD (3 MINUTES)
- Explain the workout, intended stimulus and breakdown (above).

:03–:13
GENERAL WARM-UP (10 MINUTES)
- Explain at the board and have athletes complete the work at their own pace with a 10-minute limit. It should be steady but not rushed.
- Cue throughout.
- 800-m run.
- Two rounds, 15 reps of each movement, of (first round/second round):
  - Squat therapy/PVC front squats.
  - Ring rows/strict pull-ups (banded, if necessary).
  - Push-ups/PVC shoulder presses.
  - AbMat sit-ups/hollow-body rocks.
  - Hip extensions/Supermans.

:13–:23
PULL-UP SPECIFIC WARM-UP (10 MINUTES)
If an athlete can perform 8-10 consecutive pull-ups in the warm-up, it is likely the athlete can complete the prescribed reps in the workout.

- Bar hang (30 seconds).
  - Look for: grip strength.
- 10 kipping swings.
  - Look for: tight body position.
- 10 kipping swings focusing on a big kip.
  - Look for: vertical displacement of the hips.
- 10 pull-ups (banded if necessary).
- Teach: gymnastics versus butterfly kip.
  - Allow 5 minutes for athletes to practice and refine mechanics.
  - Encourage small sets of refined movement and ensure athletes do not unduly fatigue themselves.

:23–:36
THRUSTER SPECIFIC WARM-UP (13 MINUTES)
Assess movement to determine proper workout loading.

- 60-second barbell rack-wrist stretch.
  - Allow them to come off/on tension as needed.
- 6 front squats with a pause at bottom.
  - Look for: hips pushing back to initiate.

- 6 shoulder presses with a pause overheard.
  - Look for: neutral spine.
- 6 thrusters on the coach's cadence with a reset at the rack position.
  - Look for: timing of the press.
- 6 thrusters on their own cadence.
  - Encourage them to move fast.
- Instruct athletes to add weight to reach their workout load.
  - On their own cadence, they perform 3 sets of 3 reps per set.
  - After each set, they perform 3 pull-ups.
  - Scale loads as appropriate

:36–:39
BREAK & LOGISTICS (3 MINUTES)

- Bathroom break.
- Remind athletes that additional scaling might occur during the workout.
- Review scaling options with each athlete.
- Safety check: Ensure adequate room around barbells (including for bounces after bars are dropped) and pull-up spaces (e.g., boxes to the side of a working athlete).
- Rebrief workout, flow and safety considerations.

:39–:50
WORKOUT: START AT :39 (11 MINUTES)

Cue athletes to achieve better positions while maintaining technique. Further scale the workout as needed.

- Thruster: Look for athletes who shift weight forward to the toes and press too soon (fatiguing the arms).
- Pull-up: Look for full range of motion at bottom and the top.

:50–:60
COOL-DOWN (10 MINUTES)

- Clean up equipment.
- Shoulder stretch (1 minute each side).
- Forearm "smash" (e.g., lacrosse ball) (1 minute each arm).
- Collect scores, celebrate new personal records, and exchange high fives!

WOD SCALE: FRAN

WORKOUT

Fran

21-15-9 reps of:

95-lb. thrusters

Pull-ups

Score: total time

SCALING THIS WOD

This workout is classic benchmark that allows athletes and coaches to assess progress. Fran, a couplet of gymnastics and weightlifting movements, is a relatively fast workout elite finish in less than 2 minutes.

The suggested female Rx'd weight is 65 lb. for the thruster. Either element may be modified in load. Athletes should aim to complete the workout under 10 minutes. Coaches are encouraged to use their judgment to find challenging but manageable substitutions for their athletes.

BEGINNER

21-15-9 reps of:

65-lb./45-lb. thrusters

Ring rows

- The reps remain unchanged and should be acceptable for most beginners with the reduced loads.

- The thruster weight is lowered.

- Ring rows lower the upper-body demand while still developing basic pulling strength. Adjusting the athlete's foot position to keep the body more vertical reduces the upper-body demand; choose a position that allows him or her to complete each set with no more than 2 breaks.

INTERMEDIATE

21-15-9 reps of:

95-lb./65-lb. thrusters

15-12-9

Pull-ups

- Many intermediate athletes can do this workout as prescribed.

- In cases where kipping pull-ups are a newly acquired skill, consider reducing the reps. If 8-10 consecutive pull-ups are not yet feasible, it is recommended coaches lower the volume.

LESSON PLAN: BACK SQUAT

WORKOUT
Back squat
5-5-5-5-5

Score: maximum load for a set of 5 reps

INTENDED STIMULUS
This workout is a single-modality weightlifting heavy day. Today, the sets are ascending (i.e., add weight after every set). At 5 reps per set, the workout has a slight bias toward strength-stamina versus top-end strength.

The goal is to lift the maximum load possible for a set of 5 reps while maintaining sound technique. Adequate rest (i.e., 3-5 minutes) must be taken between these sets to maximize loading.

BREAKDOWN
- The goal is to develop strength, although at 5 reps per set the loads will not be close to 1-repetition maximums.

- Athletes are expected to add load after a successful 5-rep set.

- New personal records should be attempted in the third or fourth set.

- Scaling options are modulated by load.

- Coaches should ask if any athletes are injured.

- Coaches should demonstrate the movement, including movement standards.

- Coaches should explain the score is the maximum load for a set of 5 reps.

- The load is reduced when 5 reps are not achieved or form degrades significantly.

- Suggested rest periods: 3-5 minutes between working sets.

Coaches: All parts of the class are coach led. Demonstrate each new piece before athletes perform it. Cue athletes to achieve better positions throughout each section.

:00–:03

WHITEBOARD (3 MINUTES)

- Explain the workout, intended stimulus and breakdown (above).

:03–:08

GENERAL WARM-UP (5 MINUTES)

Assess for hip, knee and ankle range of motion. Athletes might need assistance selecting an appropriate PVC pipe height.

OVER-UNDER

- Partner 1 holds a PVC pipe parallel to the ground at approximately hip height.
- Partner 2 lifts one leg at a time over the PVC, then squats and moves underneath it to return to the other side.
- Partner 2 completes 5 reps with each leg, and then the partners switch roles.
- Each person completes two turns in each role.

WALKING LUNGE STRETCH

- Athletes step out with one leg into a lunge while the hands, with interlaced fingers, reach up and to the opposite side of the front leg.
- Have the athletes stand and repeat with the opposite leg until they have completed 5 steps with each leg.

:08–:23

BACK SQUAT SPECIFIC WARM-UP (15 MINUTES)

Assess movement to determine proper workout loading.

- Have athletes partner or group together on racks set to appropriate heights.
- One athlete at a time is cued through this sequence:
  - Place the barbell on the back.
  - Brace the abdominals.
  - Step two steps back from the rack.
  - Squat to full depth.
  - Pause at the bottom.
  - Stand up aggressively.
  - Exhale at the top.
- Have each athlete repeat that sequence 4 more times on his or her own.

- Rotate new athletes in. Continue in this manner, cueing the first rep and allowing 4 independent reps, until everyone has completed a set.
  - Look for: hips initiating back and down, lumbar curve maintained and weight on the heels.
- Instruct athletes to warm up to their first working set (about 80 percent of current max).
  - They perform 3-4 sets of 5 reps per set, increasing the load after each.
  - They do not need to pause at the bottom.
- Inform athletes they must be spotted on 1 rep in one warm-up set.
  - Teach and demonstrate spotting techniques before athletes practice them.

:23–:26
BREAK & LOGISTICS (3 MINUTES)
- Bathroom break.
- Remind athletes that coaches will be cueing during lifts.
- Continue to review scaling options with each athlete.
- Safety check: Ensure adequate room around racks for bailing, and ensure athletes understand how to spot.
- Re-brief workout, flow and safety considerations.

:26–:53
WORKOUT: START WORKOUT AT :26 (27 MINUTES)
Cue athletes to better positions while maintaining technique. Reduce load when needed.

- Ensure athletes load and unload barbells safely.
- Ensure plates are clearly off the platform and will not create a hazard if a barbell is dropped.
- Make suggestions for loading based on technique displayed.

:53–:60
COOL-DOWN (7 MINUTES)
- Clean up equipment.
- Hip-flexor stretch (1 minute each leg).
- Collect scores, celebrate new personal records, and exchange high fives!

WOD SCALE: BACK SQUAT

WORKOUT

Back squat

5-5-5-5-5

Score: maximum load for a set of 5 reps

SCALING THIS WOD

This workout is a single-modality weightlifting heavy day. For today's heavy day, the sets are ascending (i.e., add weight after every set).

Regardless of experience, all athletes should find a heavy set of 5 relative to their capacity. For this workout, it is acceptable for beginner or intermediate athletes to complete more than 5 working sets if they have not yet previously established a 5-rep maximum, but coaches need to ensure the overall volume remains appropriate.

LESSON PLAN: 20-MINUTE AMRAP

WORKOUT
Complete as many rounds as possible in 20 minutes of:
Run 400 m
15 L pull-ups
205-lb. clean and jerk, 5 reps

Score: completed rounds and reps

INTENDED STIMULUS
This workout is a triplet of monostructural, gymnastics and weightlifting movements. Coaches should expect athletes to complete 4 or more rounds.

This workout taxes athletes metabolically and technically: The 400-m run elevates the heart rate, increasing the difficulty of the other two elements. L pull-ups require greater midline and pulling strength than strict pull-ups. The clean and jerk loading is intended to be moderate so the reps can be performed touch-and-go or as relatively quick singles.

BREAKDOWN
- Given the added stress from the run, the loading and reps of the L pull-ups and clean and jerk should be well within the athlete's capacity when considered independently.

- The suggested female Rx'd weight is 135 lb. for the clean and jerk.

- The scaling options include reduced volume on the run, reduced volume and load on the L pull-ups, and reduced load on the clean and jerk.

- Coaches should demonstrate each movement, including movement standards.

- Coaches should explain the workout is scored by completed rounds and reps.

- Coaches should ask if any athletes are injured.

- Athletes should aim to complete at least 4 rounds. Approximate maximum estimates of time spent on each component: 2 minutes for the run, 2 minutes for the L pull-ups and 1 minute for the clean and jerks.

Coaches: All parts of the class are coach led. Demonstrate each new piece before athletes perform it. Cue athletes to achieve better positions throughout each section.

:00–:03
WHITEBOARD (3 MINUTES)
- Explain the workout, intended stimulus and breakdown (above).

:03–:09
GENERAL WARM-UP (6 MINUTES)
If athletes are laboring on the run, struggling to perform the straight-leg raises or pull-ups, or not maintaining positioning in the deadlifts, scales are needed for the workout.

- 100-m run + 6 kip swings + 6 deadlifts (empty barbell).
- 100-m run + 6 straight-leg raises to an L + 6 deadlifts (empty barbell).
- 100-m run + 6 strict pull-ups + 6 deadlifts (empty barbell).

:09–:23
SPECIFIC CLEAN AND JERK WARM-UP (14 MINUTES)
Assess movement to determine proper workout loading.

CLEAN
- 6 deadlift-shrugs with empty barbell.
  - Look for: straight arms.
- 6 deadlift-high pulls with empty barbell.
  - Look for: bar staying close to the body.
- 6 power cleans with empty barbell.
  - Look for: proper receiving position and reset of the feet.

JERK
- 6 jump and land without barbell.
  - Look for: jumping through heels.
- 6 jump and land with hands at shoulders.
  - Look for: full hip extension.
- 6 jump and punch hands overhead.
  - Look for: timing of press after hip extension.
- 6 push jerks with empty barbell.

CLEAN AND JERK
- 6 power clean and jerks with pause after receiving the clean.
  - Teach: reset of the hands and feet.
- 12 power clean and jerks with athletes on their own cadence.
  - Look for: all major points of performance to determine for proper loading.
- Instruct athletes to work up to their workout load.
  - Athletes perform 3-4 sets of 3 reps per set, increasing the load after each set.
  - Athletes should be capable of performing 5 reps within short succession.
  - Coaches should scale loads appropriately based on movement in warm-up.

:23–30

L PULL-UP SPECIFIC WARM-UP (7 MINUTES)

Ensure athletes are prepared for the workout without being too fatigued from work in this section.

- 3 strict pull-ups (banded if necessary).
    - Remind athletes proper range of motion includes arm extension at the bottom (this will be challenging in the L pull-up).
- 3 straight-leg raises with pause in L position.
    - Teach athletes to squeeze heels together with toes pointed and legs straight.
    - Capacity displayed here will help coaches determine whether L pull-ups should be used in the workout.
- 3 L pull-ups (banded if necessary).
    - Remind athletes that the pull-up starts with the legs elevated in the L position; it is not a "kipping" rep in which the legs swing to the L position with momentum.

:30–:33

BREAK & LOGISTICS (3 MINUTES)

- Bathroom break.
- Remind athletes that additional scaling might occur during the workout.
- Review scaling options with each athlete.
- Safety check: Ensure adequate room around pull-up bars and barbells.
- Re-brief workout, flow and safety considerations.

:33–:53

WORKOUT: START AT :33 (20 MINUTES)

Cue athletes to better positions while maintaining technique. Scale workout further if needed.

- Consider scaling for athletes who do not complete the first round in about 4 minutes; scale those who take more than 5 minutes.

:53–:60

COOL DOWN (7 MINUTES)

- Clean up equipment.
- Hip-flexor stretch (1 minute each leg).
- Lat stretch (1 minute each arm).
- Collect scores and exchange high fives!

WOD SCALE: 20-MINUTE AMRAP

WORKOUT

Complete as many rounds as possible in 20 minutes of:
Run 400 m
15 L pull-ups
205-lb. clean and jerk, 5 reps

Score: completed rounds

SCALING THIS WOD

This workout is a triplet of monostructural, gymnastics and weightlifting movements. Coaches should expect athletes to complete 4 or more rounds.

The suggested female Rx'd weight is 135 lb. for the clean and jerk. One, two or all of the workout elements may be modified in volume or load. Coaches are encouraged to use their judgment for finding a challenging but manageable substitution for athletes.

BEGINNER

Complete as many rounds as possible in 20 minutes of:
Run 200 m
10 banded L pull-ups
115-lb./75-lb. clean and jerk, 5 reps

- The distance for the run has been reduced.

- The L pull-ups have been modified in reps and loading to reduce the demand on the midline and upper-body pulling muscles. The band should allow for full range of motion in proper positions.

- The clean and jerk load is lowered to allow for a relatively quick set.

INTERMEDIATE

Complete as many rounds as possible in 20 minutes of:
Run 400 m
10 L pull-ups
155-lb./105-lb. clean and jerk, 5 reps

- The L pull-ups reps have been reduced so that each round can be completed in about 2 sets.

- The clean and jerk load has been reduced to keep the intensity high.

ANATOMY AND PHYSIOLOGY FOR JOCKS

Originally published in August 2003.

Effective coaching requires efficient communication. This communication is greatly aided when coach and athlete share a terminology for both human movement and body parts.

We have developed an exceedingly simple lesson in anatomy and physiology that we believe has improved our ability to accurately and precisely motivate desired behaviors and enhanced our athletes' understanding of both movement and posture.

Basically, we ask that our athletes learn four body parts, three joints (not including the spine), and two general directions for joint movement. We cap our Anatomy and Physiology lesson with the essence of sports biomechanics distilled to three simple rules.

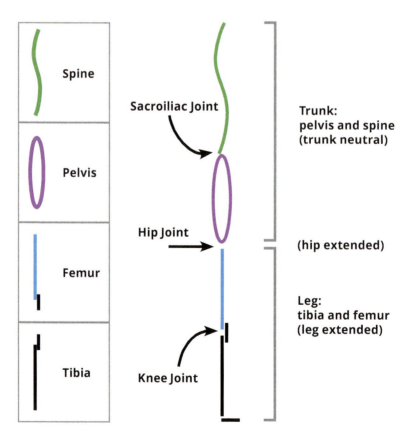

Figure 1. Essential Anatomy and Physiology.

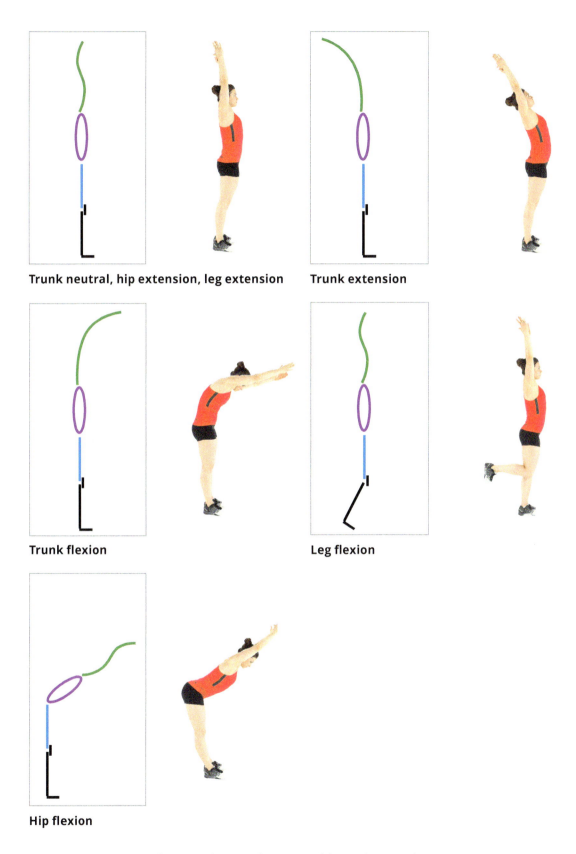

Trunk neutral, hip extension, leg extension

Trunk extension

Trunk flexion

Leg flexion

Hip flexion

Figure 2. Flexion and Extension of the Trunk, Hip, and Leg.

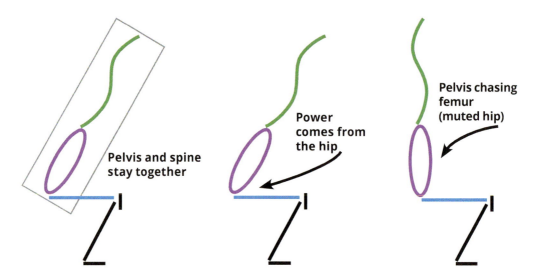

Figure 3. Midline Stabilization Versus Muted Hip.

We use a simple iconography to depict the spine, pelvis, femur, and tibia. We show that the spine has a normal "S" shape and we show where it is on the athlete's body. We similarly demonstrate the pelvis, femur, and tibia (Figure 1).

We next demonstrate the motion of three joints. First, the knee is the joint connecting tibia and femur. Second, working our way up, is the hip. The hip is the joint that connects the femur to the pelvis. Third, is the sacroiliac joint (SI joint), which connects the pelvis to the spine. (We additionally make the point that the spine is really a whole bunch of joints.)

We explain that the femur and tibia constitute "the leg" and that the pelvis and spine constitute "the trunk."

That completes our anatomy lesson–now for the physiology. We demonstrate that "flexion" is reducing the angle of a joint and that "extension" is increasing the angle of a joint.

Before covering our distillation of essential biomechanics, we test our students to see if everyone can flex and extend their knee (or "leg"), hip, spine, and sacroiliac joint (or "trunk") on cue. When it is clear that the difference between flexion and extension is understood at each joint, we cue for combinations of behaviors, for instance, "flex one leg and trunk but not your hip" (Figure 2).

Once the joints, parts, and movements are clear we offer these three tidbits of biomechanics:

- Functional movement generally weds the spine to the pelvis. The SI joint and spine were designed for small-range movement in multiple directions. Endeavor to keep the trunk tight and solid for running, jumping, squatting, throwing, cycling, etc.

- The dynamics of those movements comes from the hip–primarily extension. Powerful hip extension is certainly necessary and nearly sufficient for elite athletic capacity.

- Do not let the pelvis chase the femur instead of the spine. We refer to this as "muted hip function": the pelvis chases the femur. The hip angle remains open and is consequently powerless to extend (Figure 3).

Four parts, three joints, two motions, and three rules give our athletes and us a simple but powerful lexicon and understanding whose immediate effect is to render our athletes at once more "coachable." We could not ask for more. ▪

SQUAT CLINIC

Originally published in December 2002.

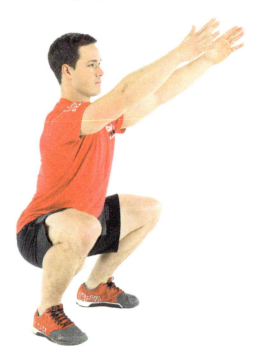

The squat is essential to your well-being. The squat can both greatly improve your athleticism and keep your hips, back, and knees sound and functioning in your senior years.

Not only is the squat not detrimental to the knees, but it is remarkably rehabilitative of cranky, damaged, or delicate knees. In fact, if you do not squat, your knees are not healthy regardless of how free of pain or discomfort you are. This is equally true of the hips and back.

The squat is no more an invention of a coach or trainer than is the hiccup or sneeze. It is a vital, natural, functional component of your being.

The squat, in the bottom position, is nature's intended sitting posture (chairs are not part of your biological makeup), and the rise from the bottom to the stand is the biomechanically sound method by which we stand up. There is nothing contrived or artificial about this movement.

Most of the world's inhabitants sit not on chairs but in a squat. Meals, ceremonies, conversation, gatherings, and defecation are all performed bereft of chairs or seats. Only in the industrialized world do we find the need for chairs, couches, benches, and stools. This comes at a loss of functionality that contributes immensely to decrepitude.

Frequently, we encounter individuals whose doctor or chiropractor has told them not to squat. In nearly every instance this is pure ignorance on the part of the practitioner. When doctors who do not like the squat are asked, "By what method should your patient get off the toilet?" they are at a loss for words.

In a similarly misinformed manner we have heard trainers and health care providers suggest that the knee should not be bent past 90 degrees. It is entertaining to ask proponents of this view to sit on the ground with their legs out in front of them and then to stand without bending the legs more than 90 degrees. It cannot be done without some grotesque bit of contrived movement. The truth is that getting up off of the floor involves a force on at least one knee that is substantially greater than the squat.

HOW TO SQUAT

Here are some valuable cues to a sound squat. Many encourage identical behaviors.

1. Start with the feet about shoulder width apart and slightly toed out.
2. Keep your head up, looking slightly above parallel.
3. Do not look down at all; ground is in the peripheral vision only.
4. Accentuate the normal arch of the lumbar curve and then pull the excess arch out with the abs.
5. Keep the midsection very tight.
6. Send your butt back and down.
7. Your knees track over the line of the foot.
8. Do not let the knees roll inside the foot. Keep as much pressure on the heels as possible.
9. Stay off the balls of the feet.
10. Delay the knees' forward travel as much as possible.
11. Lift your arms out and up as you descend.
12. Keep your torso elongated.
13. Send your hands as far away from your butt as possible.
14. In profile, the ear does not move forward during the squat; it travels straight down.
15. Do not let the squat just sink, but pull yourself down with your hip flexors.
16. Do not let the lumbar curve surrender as you settle into the bottom.
17. Stop when the fold of the hip is below the knees–break parallel with the thigh.
18. Squeeze the glutes and hamstrings and rise without any leaning forward or shifting of balance.
19. Return on the exact same path as you descended.
20. Use every bit of musculature you can; there is no part of the body uninvolved.
21. On rising, without moving the feet, exert pressure to the outside of your feet as though you were trying to separate the ground beneath you.
22. At the top of the stroke, stand as tall as you possibly can.

Our presumption is that those who counsel against the squat are either just repeating nonsense they have heard in the media or at the gym, or in their clinical practice they have encountered people who have injured themselves squatting incorrectly.

It is entirely possible to injure yourself squatting incorrectly, but it is also exceedingly easy to bring the squat to a level of safety matched by walking.

On the athletic front, the squat is the quintessential hip extension exercise, and hip extension is the foundation of all good human movement. Powerful, controlled hip extension is necessary and nearly sufficient for elite athleticism. "Necessary" in that without powerful, controlled hip extension you are not functioning anywhere near your potential. "Sufficient" in the sense that everyone we have met with the capacity to explosively open the hip could also run, jump, throw, and punch with impressive force.

Secondarily, but no less important, the squat is among those exercises eliciting a potent neuroendocrine response. This benefit is ample reason for an exercise's inclusion in your regimen.

THE AIR SQUAT

All our athletes begin their squatting with the "air squat"; that is, without any weight other than body weight. As a matter of terminology, when we refer to the "squat" we are talking about an unladen, body-weight-only squat. When we wish to refer to a weighted squat we will use the term back squat, overhead squat, or front squat, referring to those distinct weighted squats. Training with the front, back, and overhead squats before the weightless variant has been mastered retards athletic potential and compromises safety and efficacy.

When has the squat been mastered? This is a good question. It is fair to say that the squat is mastered when both technique and performance are superior. This suggests that none of the points of performance are deficient and fast multiple reps are possible. Our favorite standard for fast multiple reps would be the Tabata squat (20 seconds on/10 seconds off repeated 8 times) with the weakest of eight intervals being between 18 and 20 reps. Do not misunderstand—we are looking for 18-20 perfect squats in 20 seconds, rest for 10, and repeat seven more times for a total of eight intervals.

The most common faults to look for are surrendering of the lumbar curve at the bottom, not breaking the parallel plane with the hips, slouching in the chest and shoulders, lifting the heels, and not fully extending the hip at the top (Figure 1). Do not even think about weighted squats until none of these faults belong to you.

A relatively small angle of hip extension, while indicative of a beginner's or weak squat and caused by weak hips extensors, is not strictly considered a fault as long as the lumbar spine is neutral.

CAUSES OF A BAD SQUAT

1) Weak glute/hamstring. The glutes and hams are responsible for powerful hip extension, which is the key to the athletic performance universe.
2) Poor engagement, weak control, and no awareness of glute and hamstring. The road to powerful, effective hip extension is a three-to-five-year odyssey for most athletes.
3) Attempting to squat with quads. Leg extension dominance over hip extension is a leading obstacle to elite performance in athletes.
4) Inflexibility. Tight hamstrings are a powerful contributor to slipping into lumbar flexion–the worst fault of all.
5) Sloppy work, poor focus. This is not going to come out right by accident. It takes incredible effort. The more you work on the squat, the more awareness you develop as to its complexity.

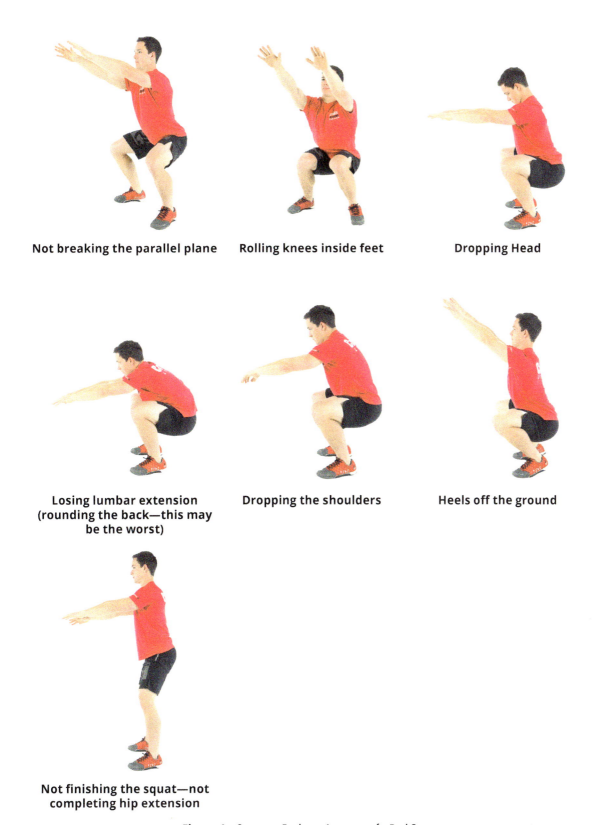

Figure 1. Common Faults or Anatomy of a Bad Squat.

TABLE 1. SQUAT TROUBLESHOOTING: COMMON FAULTS AND THERAPIES		
Faults	**Causes**	**Therapies**
Not going to parallel (not deep enough)	Weak hip extensors, laziness, quad dominance	Bottom to bottoms, bar holds, box squatting
Rolling knees inside feet	Weak adductors, weak abductors, cheat to quads	Push feet to outside of shoe, deliberately abduct (attempt to stretch floor apart beneath feet)
Dropping head	Lack of focus, weak upper back, lack of upper-back control	Bar holds, overhead squats
Losing lumbar extension	Lack of focus, tight hamstrings, cheat for balance due to weak glute/hams	Bar holds, overhead squats
Dropping shoulders	Lack of focus, weak upper back, lack of upper-back control, tight shoulders	Bar holds, overhead squats
Heels off ground	Cheat for balance due to weak glute/hams	Focus, bar holds

THERAPIES FOR COMMON FAULTS

Bar Holds: Grab a bar racked higher and closer than your normal reach at the bottom of a squat, then settle into a perfect bottom position with chest, head, hands, arms, shoulders, and back higher than usual (Figure 2). Find balance, let go, repeat closer and higher, etc. This lifts the squat (raises head, chest, shoulders, and torso), putting more load on heels and glute/hams. This immediately forces a solid bottom posture from which you have the opportunity to feel the forces required to balance in good posture. This is a reasonable shoulder stretch but not as good as the overhead squat.

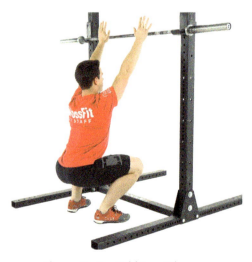

Figure 2. Bar Hold Squat Therapy.

Box Squatting: Squat to a 10-inch box, rest at the bottom without altering posture, then squeeze and rise without rocking forward. Keep a perfect posture at the bottom. This is a classic bit of technology perfected at the Westside Barbell Club.

Bottom-to-Bottoms: Stay at the bottom, come up to full extension, and quickly return to the bottom, spending much more time at the bottom than the top; for instance, sitting in the bottom for five minutes, coming up to full extension only once every five seconds (60 reps) (Figure 3). Many will avoid the bottom like the plague. You want to get down there, stay down there, and learn to like it.

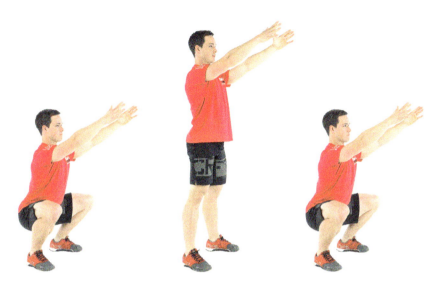

Figure 3. Bottom-to-Bottoms Squat Therapy.

Overhead Squats: Hold broomstick at snatch-grip width directly overhead, arms locked. The triangle formed by the arms and stick must stay perfectly perpendicular to the ground as you squat (Figure 4). This is a good shoulder stretch and lifts the squat. With weight, this exercise demands good balance and posture or loads become wildly unmanageable. The overhead squat is a quick punisher of sloppy technique. If shoulders are too tight, this movement will give an instant diagnosis. You can move into a doorway and find where the arms fall and cause the stick to bang into the doorway. Lift the arms, head, chest, back, and hip enough to travel up and down without hitting the doorway. Over time, work to move the feet closer and closer to the doorway without hitting it. The broomstick foundation is critical to learning the snatch–the world's fastest lift.

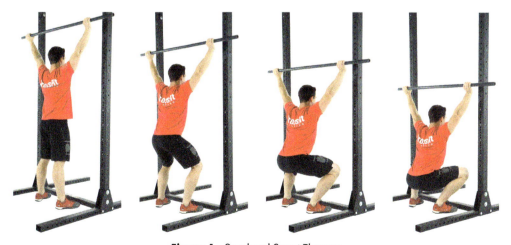

Figure 4. Overhead Squat Therapy.

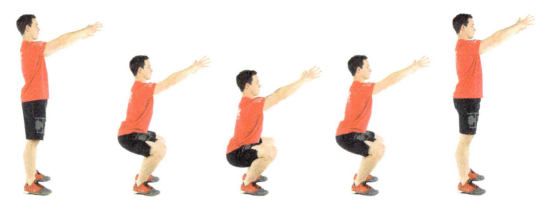

Figure 5. Air Squat.

AIR SQUAT

- Maintain the arch in the back
- Look straight ahead
- Keep weight on heels
- Reach the full range of motion (i.e., below parallel)
- Keep the chest high
- Keep the midsection tight

The squat is essential to human movement, a proven performance enhancer and a gateway movement to the best exercise in strength and conditioning.

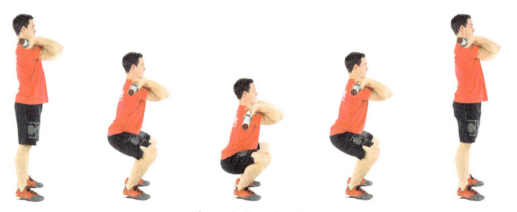

Figure 6. Front Squat.

FRONT SQUAT

- Bar rests on chest and shoulders with loose grip–"racked"
- The mechanics are otherwise like the air squat

The hardest part of the front squat might be the rack position. Practice until you can get the bar and hands in the proper position. Handstands help. This one will force shoulder and wrist flexibility. ■

THE OVERHEAD SQUAT

Originally published in August 2005.

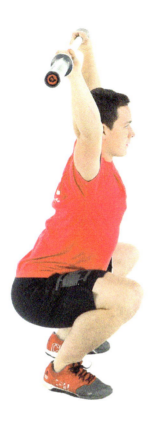

The overhead squat is the ultimate core exercise, the heart of the snatch, and peerless in developing effective athletic movement.

This functional gem trains for efficient transfer of energy from large to small body parts–the essence of sport movement. For this reason it is an indispensable tool for developing speed and power.

The overhead squat also demands and develops functional flexibility, and it similarly develops the squat by amplifying and cruelly punishing faults in squat posture, movement, and stability.

The overhead squat is to midline control, stability, and balance what the clean and snatch are to power–unsurpassed.

Ironically, the overhead squat is exceedingly simple yet universally nettlesome for beginners. There are three common obstacles to learning the overhead squat. The first is the scarcity of skilled instruction—outside the weightlifting community most instruction on the overhead squat is laughably, horribly wrong—dead wrong. The second is a weak squat—you need to have a rock-solid squat to learn the overhead squat. The third obstacle is starting with too much weight–you have not a snowball's chance in hell of learning the overhead squat with a bar. You will need to use a length of dowel or PVC pipe; use anything over 5 lb. to learn this move and your overhead squat will be stillborn.

LEARNING THE OVERHEAD SQUAT

1) Start only when you have a strong squat and use a dowel or PVC pipe, not a weight. You should be able to maintain a rock-bottom squat with your back arched, head and eyes forward, and body weight predominantly on your heels for several minutes as a prerequisite to the overhead squat. Even a 15-lb. training bar is way too heavy to learn the overhead squat (Figure 1).

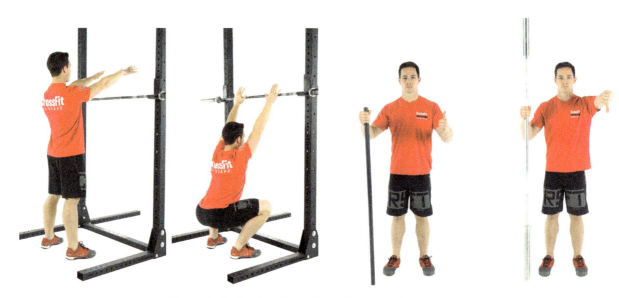

Figure 1. An Overhead Squat Depends on a Proficient Air Squat.

2) Learn locked-arm "dislocates" or "pass-throughs" with the dowel. You want to be able to move the dowel nearly 360 degrees, starting with the dowel down and at arms' length in front of your body, and then moving it in a wide arc until it comes to rest down and behind you without bending your arms at any point in its travel. Start with a grip wide enough to easily pass through, and then repeatedly bring the hands in closer until passing through presents a moderate stretch of the shoulders (Figure 2). This is your training grip.

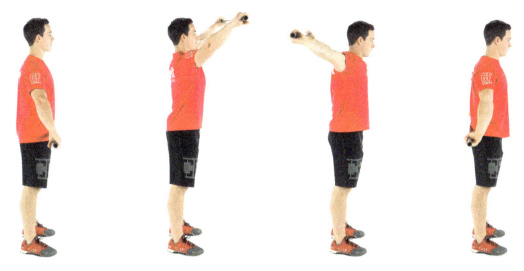

Figure 2. Shoulder Dislocates to Determine Grip Width.

3) Be able to perform the pass-through at the top, the bottom, and everywhere in between while descending into the squat. Practice by stopping at several points on the path to the bottom, hold, and gently, slowly, swing the dowel from front to back, again, with locked arms. At the bottom of each squat, slowly bring the dowel back and forth moving from front to back (Figure 3).

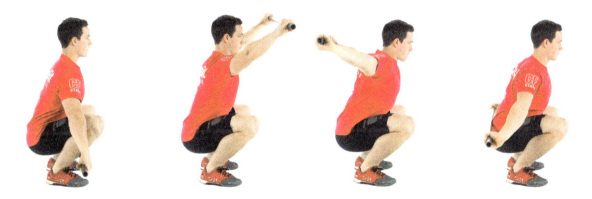

Figure 3. Shoulder Dislocates Throughout the Overhead Squat Range of Motion.

4) Learn to find the frontal plane with the dowel from every position in the squat. Practice this with your eyes closed. You want to develop a keen sense of where the frontal plane is located. This is the same drill as Step 3 but this time you are bringing the dowel to a stop in the frontal plane and holding briefly with each pass-through (Figure 4). Have a training partner check to see if at each stop the dowel is in the frontal plane.

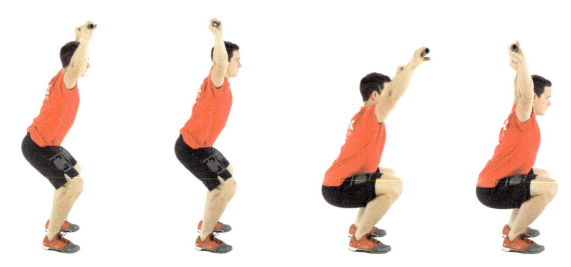

Figure 4. Shoulder Dislocates Stopping in the Frontal Plane.

5) Start the overhead squat by standing tall with the dowel held as high as possible in the frontal plane (Figure 5). You want to start with the dowel directly overhead, not behind you, or, worse yet, even a little bit in front.

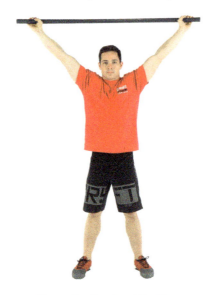

Figure 5. Overhead Position.

6) Very slowly lower to the bottom of the squat, keeping the dowel in the frontal plane the entire time (Figure 6). Have a training partner watch from your side to make sure that the dowel does not move forward or backward as you squat to the bottom. Moving slightly behind the frontal plane is acceptable, but forward is dead wrong. If you cannot keep the dowel from coming forward your grip might be too narrow. The dowel will not stay in the frontal plane automatically; you will have to pull it back very deliberately as you descend (particularly if your chest comes forward).

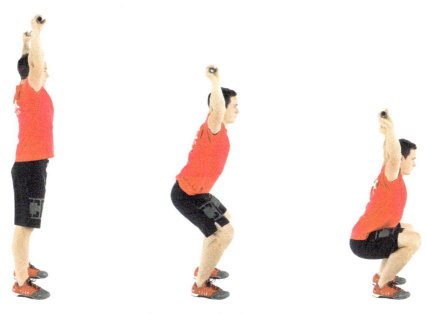

Figure 6. Overhead Squat.

7) Practice the overhead squat regularly and increase load in tiny increments. We can put a 2.5-lb. plate on the dowel, then a 5, then a 5 and a 2.5, and then a 10. Next use a 15-lb. training bar, but only while maintaining perfect form (Figure 7). There is no benefit to adding weight if the dowel, and later the bar, cannot be kept in the frontal plane.

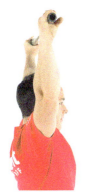 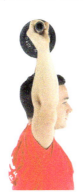 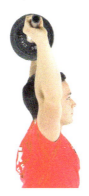 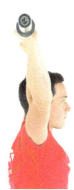

Figure 7. Increasing Weight when Learning the Overhead Squat.

With practice, you will be able to bring your hands closer together and still keep the bar in the frontal plane. Ultimately you can develop enough control and flexibility to descend to a rock-bottom squat with your feet together and hands together without the dowel coming forward. Practicing for this is a superb warm-up and cool-down drill and stretch.

The overhead squat develops core control by punishing any forward wobble of the load with an enormous and instant increase in the moment about the hip and back. When the bar is held perfectly overhead and still, which is nearly impossible, the overhead squat does not present greater load on the hip or back, but moving too fast, along the wrong line of action, or wiggling can bring even the lightest loads down like a house of cards. You have two, and only two, safe options for bailing out–dumping the load forward and stepping or falling backward, or dumping backward and stepping or falling forward. Both are safe and easy. Lateral escapes are not an option.

The difference between your overhead squat and your back or front squat is a solid measure of your midline stability and control and the precision of your squatting posture and line of action. Improving and developing your overhead squat will fix faults not visible in the back and front squat.

As your max overhead, back, and front squat each rise, their relative measure reveals much about your developing potential for athletic movement.

An average of your max back and front squat is an excellent measure of your core, hip, and leg strength. Your max overhead squat is an excellent measure of your core stability and control and ultimately your ability to generate effective and efficient athletic power.

Your max overhead squat will always be a fraction of the average of your max back and front squat but, ideally, with time, they should converge rather than diverge (Figure 8).

Should they diverge, you are developing hip and core strength, but your capacity to efficiently apply power distally is reduced. In athletic pursuits you might be prone to injury. Should they converge, you are developing useful strength and power that can be successfully applied to athletic movements.

The functional application or utility of the overhead squat might not be readily apparent, but there are many real-world occurrences where objects high enough to get under are too heavy or not free enough to be jerked or pressed overhead yet can be elevated by first lowering your hips until your arms can be locked and then squatting upward.

Once developed, the overhead squat is a thing of beauty–a masterpiece of expression in control, stability, balance, efficient power, and utility. Get on it.

A: The torso's angle of inclination above horizontal. As a squat matures this angle increases. The squat becomes more upright as the athlete's strength and neural "connectedness" to the posterior chain increase. Lower angles of inclination are created in an attempt to cantilever away from a weak posterior chain and onto the quadriceps. While technically correct, the lower angle is mechanically disadvantaged, particularly in loaded variations.

90-A: This is the angle of rotation of the arms, at the shoulders, past overhead. The lower A is, the greater the rotation, 90-A, required of the shoulders to keep the bar in the frontal plane. The larger 90-A is, the wider the grip required to allow the shoulders to rotate to keep the bar in the frontal plane. Ultimately the connectedness/strength of the posterior chain will determine the width of the grip, elevation of the squat, and degree of rotation of the shoulders. Maturity and quality of the squat are determinants of all of the mechanics of the overhead squat.

g: These lines mark horizontal.

f: This line defines the frontal plane. It divides the athlete's front half from back half. In the squat (as with most weightlifting movements), the athlete endeavors to keep the load in this plane. If a load deviates substantially from this plane the athlete has to bring the load back, which in turn pulls the athlete off balance.

b: This is roughly the position for a back or front squat.

a: This is the position for the overhead squat. With perfect stability, movement, and alignment this position does not increase the moment about the hip or back. The difference in an athlete's strength when squatting here, overhead, as opposed to Position b, the back or front squat, is a perfect measure of instability in the torso, legs, or shoulders; improper line of action in the shoulders, hips, or legs, and; weak or flawed posture in the squat.

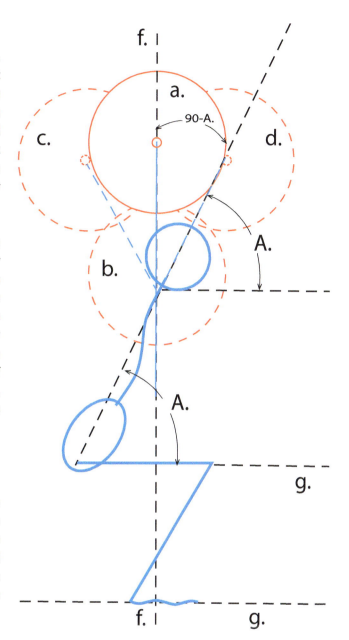

Figure 8. Relative Angles and Bar Positioning in Squat Variations.

c: This position has the load behind the frontal plane. It can actually decrease the moment on the hip and back. As long as balance is maintained, the position is strong.

d: This is a fatal flaw in the overhead squat. Even slight movement in this direction greatly increases the moment in the hip and back. Moving in this direction with even a small load can collapse the squat like a house of cards. ∎

SHOULDER PRESS, PUSH PRESS, PUSH JERK

Originally published in January 2003.

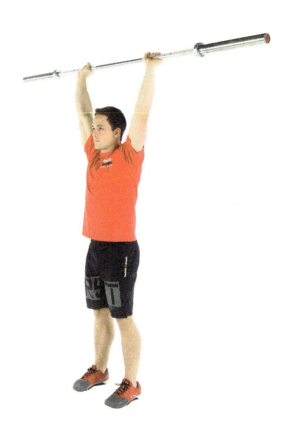

Learning the progression of lifts that moves from the shoulder press (Figure 1) to the push press (Figure 2) to the push jerk (Figure 3) has long been a CrossFit staple. This progression offers the opportunity to acquire some essential motor recruitment patterns found in sport and life (functionality) while greatly improving strength in the "power zone" and upper body. In terms of power zone and functional recruitment patterns, the push press and push jerk have no peer among other presses such as the "king" of upper-body lifts, the bench press. As the athlete moves from shoulder press to push press to push jerk, the importance of core-to-extremity muscle recruitment is learned and reinforced. This concept alone would justify the practice and training of these lifts. Core-to-extremity muscular recruitment is foundational to the effective and efficient performance of athletic movement.

The most common errors in punching, jumping, throwing, and a multitude of other athletic movements typically express themselves as a violation of this concept. Because good athletic movement begins at the core and radiates to the extremities, core strength is absolutely essential to athletic success. The region of the body from which these movements emanate, the core, is often referred to as the "power zone." The muscle groups comprising the "power zone" include the hip flexors, hip extensors (glutes and hams), spinal erectors, and quadriceps.

These lifts are enormous aids to developing the power zone. Additionally, the advanced elements of the progression, the push press and jerk, train for and develop power and speed. Power and speed are "king" in sport performance. Coupling force with velocity is the very essence of power and speed. Some of our favorite and most developmental lifts lack this quality. The push press and jerk are performed explosively–that is the hallmark of speed and power training. Finally, mastering this progression gives ideal opportunity to detect and eliminate a postural/mechanical fault that plagues more athletes than not–the pelvis "chasing" the leg during hip flexion (Figure 4). This fault needs to be searched out and destroyed. The push press performed under great stress is the perfect tool to conjure up this performance wrecker so it can be eliminated.

SHOULDER PRESS

SET-UP:	Take the bar from supports or clean to a racked position. The bar sits on the shoulders with the grip slightly wider than shoulder width. The elbows are below and in front of bar. The stance is approximately hip width.
PRESS:	Press the bar to a position directly overhead. The head must accommodate the bar.

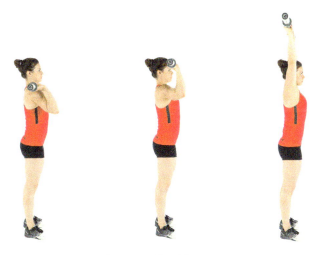

Figure 1. Shoulder Press.

PUSH PRESS

SET-UP:	The set-up is the same as the shoulder press.
DIP:	Initiate the dip by bending the hips and knees while keeping the torso upright. The dip will be only a couple of inches.
DRIVE:	With no pause at the bottom of the dip, the hips and legs are forcefully extended.
PRESS:	As the hips and legs complete extension, the shoulders and arms forcefully press the bar overhead until the arms are fully extended.

PUSH JERK

SET-UP:	The set-up is the same as the shoulder press and push press.
DIP:	The dip is identical to the push press.
DRIVE:	The drive is identical to the push press.
PRESS UNDER:	This time instead of just pressing, you press and dip a second time simultaneously, catching the bar in a partial squat with the arms fully extended overhead.
FINISH:	Stand to fully erect with bar directly overhead, identical to the finish position in the push press and shoulder press.

THE ROLE OF THE ABS IN THE OVERHEAD LIFTS

Athletically, the abdominals' primary role is midline stabilization, not trunk flexion. They are critical to swimming, running, cycling, and jumping, but never is their stabilizing role more critical than when attempting to drive loads overhead, and, of course, the heavier the load, the more critical the abs' role becomes. We train our athletes to think of every exercise as an ab exercise but in the overhead lifts it is absolutely essential to do so. It is easy to see when an athlete is not sufficiently engaging the abs in an overhead press—the body arches so as to push the hips, pelvis, and stomach ahead of the bar. Constant vigilance is required of every lifter to prevent and correct this postural deformation.

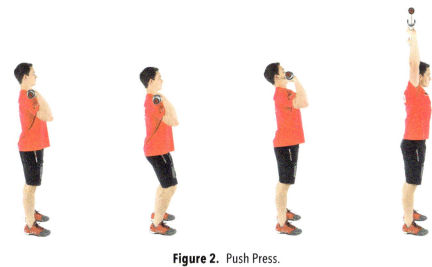

Figure 2. Push Press.

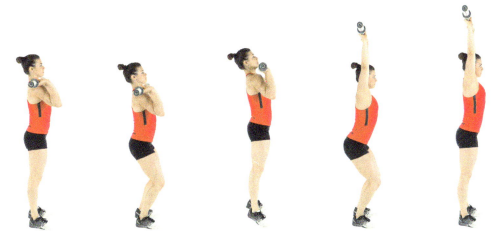

Figure 3. Push Jerk.

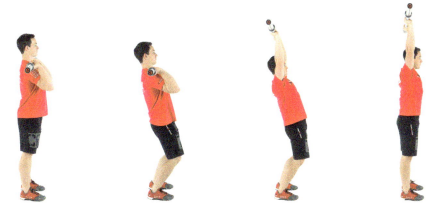

Figure 4. The Muted Hip in the Dip Phase.

SUMMARY

From shoulder press to push jerk the movements become increasingly more athletic, functional, and suited to heavier loads. The progression also increasingly relies on the power zone. In the shoulder press, the power zone is used for stabilization only. In the push press the power zone provides not only stability but also the primary impetus in both the dip and drive. In the push jerk the power zone is called on for the dip, drive, second dip, and squat. The role of the hip is increased in each exercise.

With the push press you will be able to drive overhead as much as 30 percent more weight than with the shoulder press. The push jerk will allow you to drive as much as 30 percent more overhead than you would with the push press.

In effect the hip is increasingly recruited through the progression of lifts to assist the arms and shoulders in raising loads overhead. After mastering the push jerk you will find that it will unconsciously displace the push press as your method of choice when going overhead.

The second dip on the push jerk will become lower and lower as you both master the technique and increase the load. At some point in your development, the loads will become so substantial that the upper body cannot contribute but a fraction to the movement, at which point the catch becomes very low and an increasing amount of the lift is accomplished by the overhead squat.

On both the push press and jerk, the "dip" is critical to the entire movement. The stomach is held very tightly and the resultant turnaround from dip to drive is sudden, explosive, and violent.

TRY THESE

1) Start with 95 lb. and push press or push jerk 15 straight repetitions, rest 30 seconds, and repeat for total of 5 sets of 15 repetitions each. Go up in weight only when you can complete all 5 sets with only 30 seconds of rest between each and do not pause in any set.

2) Repetition 1: shoulder press, Repetition 2: push press, Repetition 3: push jerk. Repeat until shoulder press is impossible, then continue until push press is impossible, then five more push jerks. Start with 95 lb. and go up only when the total repetitions exceed 30. ▪

THE DEADLIFT

Originally published in August 2003.

The deadlift is unrivaled in its simplicity and impact while unique in its capacity for increasing head-to-toe strength.

Regardless of whether your fitness goals are to "rev up" your metabolism, increase strength or lean body mass, decrease body fat, rehabilitate your back, improve athletic performance, or maintain functional independence as a senior, the deadlift is a marked shortcut to that end.

To the detriment of millions, the deadlift is infrequently used and seldom seen either by most of the exercising public and/or, believe it or not, by athletes.

It might be that the deadlift's name has scared away the masses; its older name, "the healthlift," was a better choice for this perfect movement.

In its most advanced application the deadlift is prerequisite to, and a component of, "the world's fastest lift," the snatch, and "the world's most powerful lift," the clean, but it is also, quite simply, no more than the safe and sound approach by which any object should be lifted from the ground.

The deadlift, being no more than picking a thing off the ground, keeps company with standing, running, jumping, and throwing for functionality but imparts quick and prominent athletic advantage like no other exercise. Not until the clean, snatch, and squat are well developed will the athlete again find as useful a tool for improving general physical ability.

The deadlift's primal functionality, whole-body nature, and mechanical advantage with large loads suggest its strong neuroendocrine impact, and for most athletes the deadlift delivers such a quick boost in general strength and sense of power that its benefits are easily understood.

If you want to get stronger, improve your deadlift. Driving your deadlift up can nudge your other lifts upward, especially the Olympic lifts.

Fear of the deadlift abounds, but like fear of the squat, it is groundless. No exercise or regimen will protect the back from the potential injuries of sport and life or the certain ravages of time like the deadlift (Table 1).

We recommend deadlifting at near-max loads once per week or so and maybe one other time at loads that would be insignificant at low reps. Be patient and learn to celebrate small, infrequent bests.

The deadlift keeps company with standing, running, jumping, and throwing for functionality but imparts quick and prominent athletic advantage like no other exercise."

–COACH GLASSMAN

Major benchmarks would certainly include body-weight, twice-body-weight, and three-times-body-weight deadlifts, representing "beginning," "good," and "great" deadlifts respectively.

For us, the guiding principles of proper technique rest on three pillars: orthopedic safety, functionality, and mechanical advantage. Concerns for orthopedic stresses and limited functionality are behind our rejection of stances wider than hip to shoulder width. While acknowledging the remarkable achievements of many powerlifters with the super-wide deadlift stance, we feel that its limited functionality (we cannot safely, walk, clean, or snatch from "out there") and the increased resultant forces on the hip from wider stances warrant only infrequent and moderate to light exposures to wider stances.

Experiment and work regularly with alternate, parallel, and hook grips. Explore carefully and cautiously variances in stance, grip width, and even plate diameter—each variant uniquely stresses the margins of an all-important functional movement. This is an effective path to increased hip capacity.

Consider each of the following cues to a sound deadlift. Many motivate identical behaviors, yet each of us responds differently to different cues.

- Natural stance with feet under hips.
- Symmetrical grip whether parallel, hook, or alternate.
- Hands placed where arms will not interfere with legs while pulling from the ground.
- Bar above the knot of the shoelaces.
- Shoulders slightly forward of bar.
- Inside of elbows facing one another.
- Chest up and inflated.
- Abs tight.
- Arms locked and not pulling.
- Shoulders pinned back and down.
- Lats and triceps contracted and pressing against one another.
- Keep your weight on your heels.
- Bar stays close to legs and essentially travels straight up and down.
- Torso's angle of inclination remains constant while bar is below the knees.
- Gaze straight ahead.
- Shoulders and hips rise at same rate when bar is below the knees.
- Arms remain perpendicular to ground until lockout.

TABLE 1. TRANSCRIPT OF A CONVERSATION BETWEEN A DOCTOR AND COACH GLASSMAN	
Doc:	Many of my patients shouldn't be doing the deadlift.
Coach:	Which ones are those, Doc?
Doc:	Many are elderly, marginally ambulatory, and frail/feeble and osteoporotic.
Coach:	Doc, would you let such a patient, let's say an old woman, walk to the store to get cat food?
Doc:	Sure, if the walk weren't too far, I'd endorse it.
Coach:	All right, suppose after walking home she came up to the front door and realized that her keys were in her pocket. Is she medically cleared to set the bag down, get her keys out of her pocket, unlock the door, pick the bag back up, and go in?
Doc:	Of course, that's essential activity.
Coach:	As I see it, the only difference between us is that I want to show her how to do this "essential activity" safely and soundly and you don't.
Doc:	I see where you're going. Good point.
Coach:	Doc, we haven't scratched the surface.

DEADLIFT
- Look straight ahead.
- Keep the back arched.
- Arms do not pull; they are just straps.
- Bar travels along legs.
- Push through the heels.

The deadlift, like the squat, is an essential functional movement and carries a potent hormonal punch. This is core training like no other.

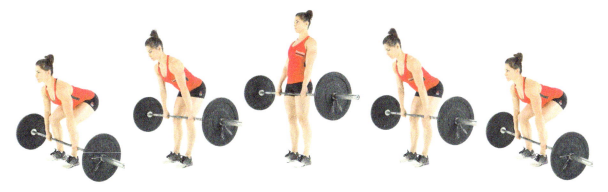

Figure 1. The Deadlift.

SUMO DEADLIFT HIGH PULL

- Start with bar at mid-shin.
- Wide, "sumo" stance.
- Take narrow grip on bar.
- Look straight ahead.
- Keep back arched.
- Pull with hips and legs only until both are at full extension.
- Aggressively open hip fully.
- Powerfully shrug.
- Immediately pull with arms to continue the upward travel of the bar.
- Keep the elbows as far above your hands as possible.
- Bring the bar right up under the chin briefly.
- Lower to hang.
- Lower to mid-shin.

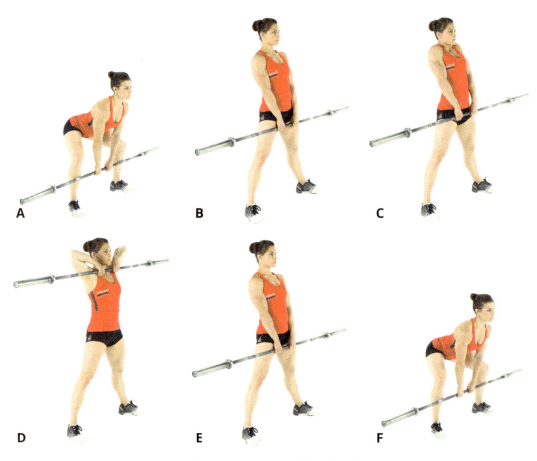

Figure 2. Sumo Deadlift High Pull.

For range of motion, line of action, and length and speed of action, the sumo deadlift high pull is a great conjugate to the thruster. At low loads this is our favorite substitute for Concept2 rowing. ∎

MEDICINE-BALL CLEANS

Originally published in September 2004.

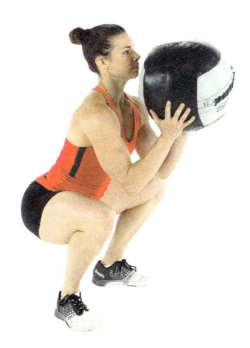

The clean and jerk and the snatch, the Olympic lifts, present the toughest learning challenge in all of weight training. Absent these lifts, there are no complex movements found in the weight room. By contrast, the average collegiate gymnast has learned hundreds of movements at least as complex, difficult, and nuanced as the clean or snatch. In large part because most weight training is exceedingly simple, learning the Olympic lifts is, for too many athletes, a shock of frustration and incompetence.

Sadly, many coaches, trainers, and athletes have avoided these movements precisely because of their technical complexity. Ironically, but not surprisingly, the technical complexity of the quick lifts exactly contains the seeds of their worth; that is, they simultaneously demand and develop strength, power, speed, flexibility, coordination, agility, balance, and accuracy.

When examining the reasons offered for not teaching the Olympic lifts we cannot help but suspect that the lifts' detractors have no first-hand (real) experience with them. We want to see someone, anyone, do a technically sound clean or snatch at any weight and then offer a rationale for the movement's restricted applicability. Were they dangerous or inappropriate for any particular population, we would find coaches intimate with the lifts articulating the nature of their inappropriateness. We do not.

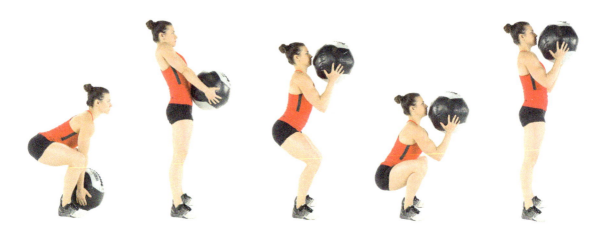

Figure 1. Medicine-Ball Clean.

At CrossFit, everyone learns the Olympic lifts—that is right, everyone.

We review here the bad rap hung on the Olympic lifts because we have made exciting progress working past the common misconceptions and fears surrounding their introduction, execution, and applicability to general populations. The medicine-ball clean has been integral to our successes.

The Dynamax medicine ball is a soft, large, pillowy ball that ranges in weight from 4 to 30 lb. available in increments. It is nonthreatening, even friendly.

Working with Dynamax balls, we introduce the starting position and posture of the deadlift, then the lift itself. In a matter of minutes we then shift our efforts to front squatting with the ball. After a little practice with the squat we move to the clean. (A similar approach is used to teach the shoulder press, push press, and push jerk.)

The clean is then reduced to "pop the hip and drop–catch it in a squat" and it is done. The devil is in the details, but the group is cleaning in five minutes. It is a legitimate, functional clean. More so even than cleaning with a bar, the medicine-ball clean might in fact have clearer application to heaving a bag of cement into a pickup or hucking up a toddler to put in a car seat.

The faults universal to lifting initiates are all there in as plain sight with the ball as with the bar. Any subtleties of matured and modern bar technique not possible with the ball are not immediate concerns, and their absence is plainly justified by the imparted understanding that this is functional stuff and applicable to all objects we might desire to heave from ground to chest.

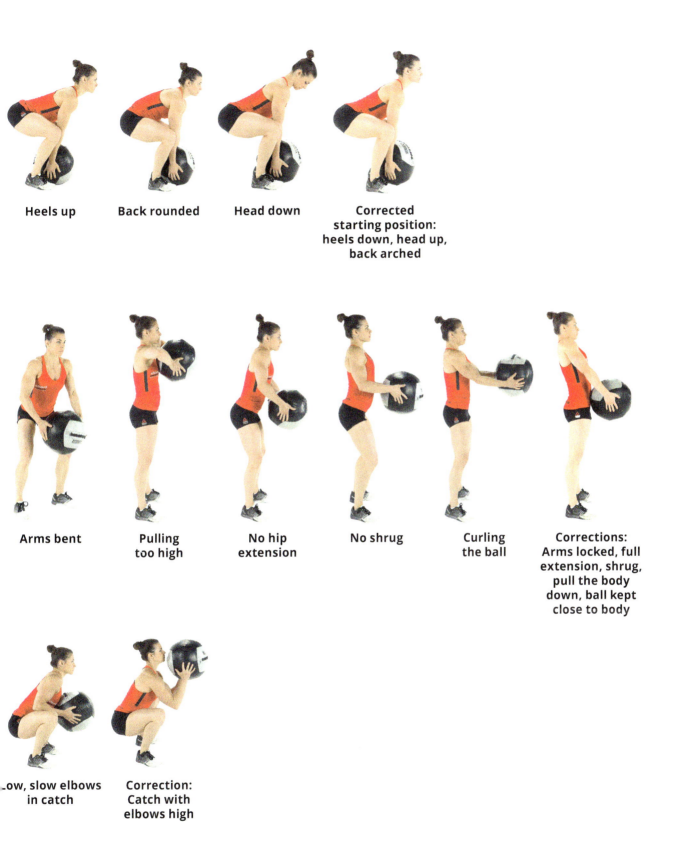

Figure 2. Medicine-Ball Clean Common Faults and Corrections.

In a group of mixed capacities the newbies get the light balls and the veterans get the heavy ones. In 30-rep doses whoever ends up with the 30-lb. ball is going to get a workout regardless of his or her abilities. The heavier balls impart a nasty wallop far beyond the same work done with a bar or dumbbell of equal weight; considerable additional effort is expended adducting the arms, which is required to "pinch" the ball and keep it from slipping.

We use the medicine-ball clean in warm-ups and cool-downs to reinforce the movement, and the results are clearly manifest in the number and rate of personal records we are seeing in bar cleans with all our athletes. Yes, the benefit transfers to the bar—even for our better lifters!

In the duration of a warm-up there are uncountable opportunities to weed out bad mechanics. Pulling with the arms, not finishing hip extension, failing to shrug, pulling too high, lifting the heels in the first pull, curling the ball, losing back extension, looking down, catching high then squatting, slow dropping under, slow elbows—all the faults are there (Figure 2).

With several weeks' practice, a group will go from "spastic" to a precision medicine-ball drill team in perfect sync. In fact, that is how we conduct the training effort.

We put the athletes in a small circle, put the best clean available in the center as leader, and ask the athletes to mirror the center. Screw-ups are clearly evident by being in postures or positions out of sync. Attention is riveted on a good model while duplicating the movement in real time. The time required for "paralysis through analysis" is wonderfully not there (Figure 2). Thinking becomes doing.

Individuals generally impervious to verbal cues become self-correcting of faults made apparent by watching and comparing to others. It is not uncommon for shouts of correction to be lobbed across the circle from participant to participant. Coaching cues and discussion are reduced to the minimum and essential as the process is turned into a child's game of "follow the leader."

Where this becomes "dangerous," "bad for the joints," "too technical to learn," or any other nonsense routinely uttered about weightlifting, we do not know. ∎

THE GLUTE-HAM DEVELOPER (GHD)

Adapted from Coach Glassman's March 18, 2007, L1 lecture in Raleigh, North Carolina.

Our definition of core strength is midline stabilization. In profile, there is a reference line that trisects the spine and bisects the pelvis. Midline stabilization is the ability to maintain rigidity, stability, and a lack of deflection about that line (Figure 1). This translates to improved efficiency and performance and greater power output.

It is critical to the deadlift, to the laden squat, to the shoulder press, and to any sport. In a swimmer's stroke—when the left leg kicks and right arm pulls—if the torso deviates to one side, you lose energy. Energy is lost in its deflection, whether throwing a punch, riding a bicycle, or squatting. The abdominals, with the hip flexors, control one side of the torso, with the hip extensors and erectors involved on the other side.

However, what we have in modern physical culture is an excessive awareness and focus on the anterior and not on the posterior. As a culture of athletes and non-athletes alike, we are unfortunately frontally fixated. Pecs—what about the rhomboids? Abs—what about the erectors? Quads—what about the glute-hamstring? And for the best of functional movement—punch, jump, throw, run—the impetus comes out of the posterior.

We see communities where there is a very deliberate and concerted effort to minimize hip-flexor involvement in exercise. And yet, by insertion and origin, by mechanical position and advantage, and just kinematically, the hip flexors, have several times the contraction capacity that is estimated of the abdominals. All of it: hip extensors, hip flexors, trunk flexors, and extensors are essential to midline stabilization. The abdominals are just one part of the story.

For core strength (midline stabilization), we are talking about static control. We do not want this relationship of spine to pelvis deflecting. Nevertheless, a lot of the commonly used "core" movements involve dynamic movements: the crunch is a very deliberate flexion of the trunk. Conversely, when we deadlift, we very deliberately hold that relationship static.

What is amazing is how many communities that are regularly involved in physical training (PT) have 1) almost no effort focused on hip extension and 2) almost no awareness of the spine-to-

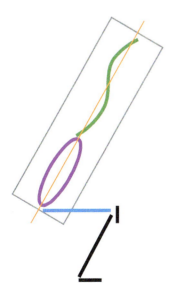

Figure 1. Midline Stabilization.

pelvis relationship. About the only thing that we see them paying attention to is dynamic trunk-flexion work. There is no trunk-extension work, no hip-extension work, and hip flexion is deliberately limited. Some of these communities also have problems with chronic back injury, which comes at no surprise. If there is anything to "muscle balance," it makes sense. In how many communities are they doing an equal number of deadlifts and squats to their sit-ups? Most of the military/law-enforcement PT is completely devoid of full-range-of-motion hip extension. Rucking, running, jumping jacks—all will not do it. The run, pull-up, sit-up, push-up, lather-rinse-repeat PT has no real good core movement. The crunch does not count.

While a cumbersome and space-taking piece of gear, the GHD has been essential to our work. We have four of them in 2,500 square feet, so one every 600 feet. We use the GHD for four exercises to heighten awareness and develop capacity at midline stabilization. The punchline to the story is that static contractions that stabilize the midsection are the most important and functional (powerful) muscular contractions in that region. Static contractions for midline stabilization are the best ab exercises known. No amount of crunches are ever going to get you to the same end point as the L-sit, overhead squat, deadlift, etc.

What we suspect is that if you could sequentially fire the abs with the same force in any kind of dynamic pattern, you would have the ability to seriously injure your spine. If you could ever crunch with the same force that you can stabilize, you would be able to break your back at will. We have come hardwired unable to do that—that is my guess.

The movements are presented in the order in which they should be developed in a client. The first thing is a simple hip extension: articulate at the hip only, maintaining the distance from xiphoid process to pubic bone. There is no shortening of the trunk. There is no trunk flexion, just hip extension and flexion while maintaining midline stabilization. The erectors are being used statically, and the primary movers here are glutes and hamstrings working concentrically and eccentrically. Be careful such that the client's femur is on the pad and the pelvis is free. If the pelvis is trapped, the athlete will not be able to hold the lumbar curve. The hip extension is static in the trunk and dynamic in the hip (Figures 2 and 3).

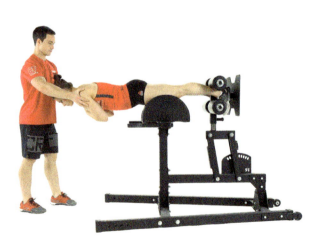

Figure 2. Trainers Can Provide Assistance for Hip Extensions Until Capacity Is Developed.

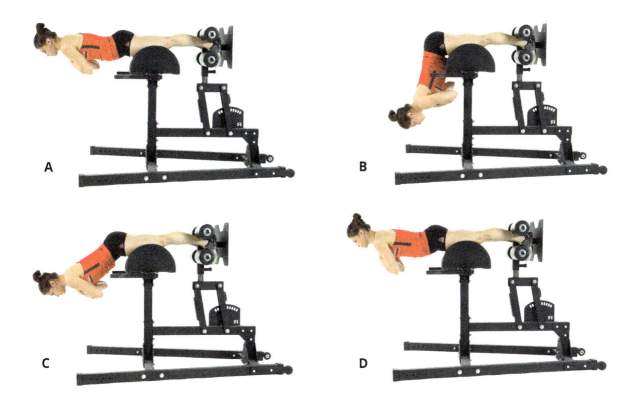

Figure 3. GHD Hip Extension.

Not only is this movement exceedingly safe, but it is also incredibly rehabilitative of the lower back. Even people with near-acute lower-back injury can do this, but ensure there is no flexion in the torso. With the capacity to do 25-30 consecutive repetitions without momentum, they will find there is substantial mitigation in whatever was bothering them. This is a milder stimulus to that region than a moderate-weight deadlift. An air squat and an insignificant-load deadlift combined with this movement create a great launching point. It is a critical part of our beginning efforts with our clients regardless of age.

Once a client has shown some competence here (25-30 consecutive reps), the next movement is the back extension. The pad has to be adjusted such that it is under the pelvis. In this movement, the athlete deliberately surrenders the lumbar curve, thereby engaging in trunk flexion and extension. The erectors are now working dynamically, with the glute and hamstring working statically or isometrically. We are doing it controlled—not bouncing, not flopping. We are doing it initially unladen (Figure 4).

When there is proven capacity in the back extension (25-30 consecutive reps), we move on to the hip-and-back extension. The pad is adjusted back to the setting used for hip extension. Starting from the bottom, extended in the spine, full flexion in the hip, the pelvis first lifts followed by a wave of contraction from lumbar

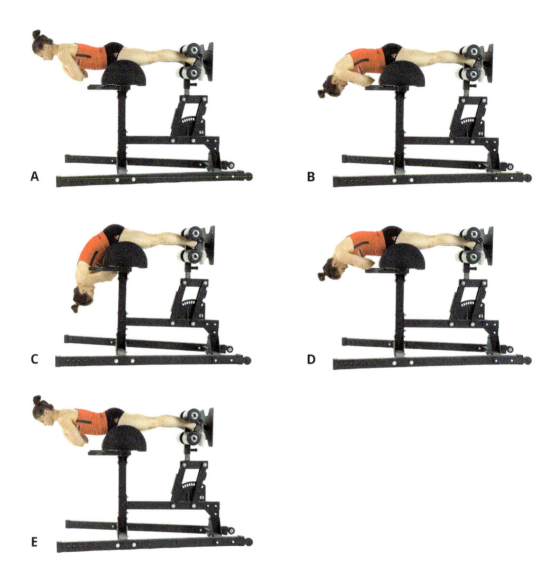

Figure 4. GHD Back Extension.

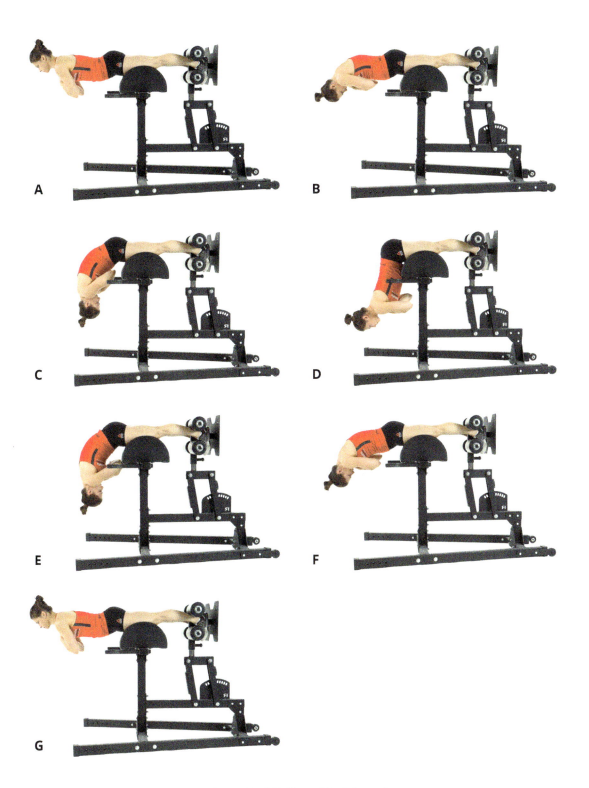

A

B

C

D

E

F

G

Figure 5. GHD Hip-and-Back Extension.

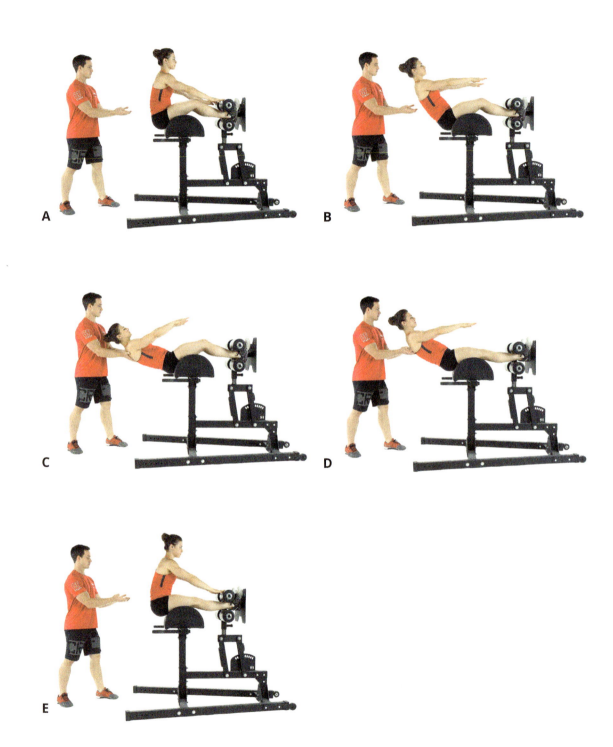

Figure 6. Trainers Should Initially Spot Clients and Shorten the
Range of Motion in the GHD Sit-up.

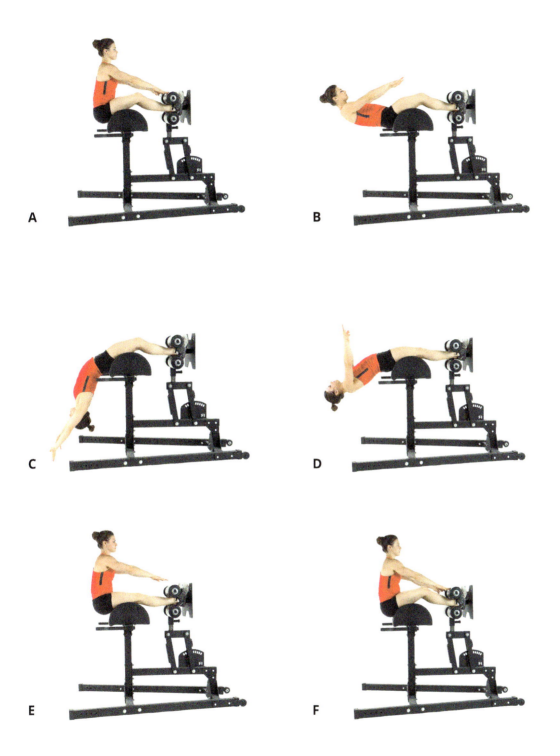

A

B

C

D

E

F

Figure 7. GHD Sit-up.

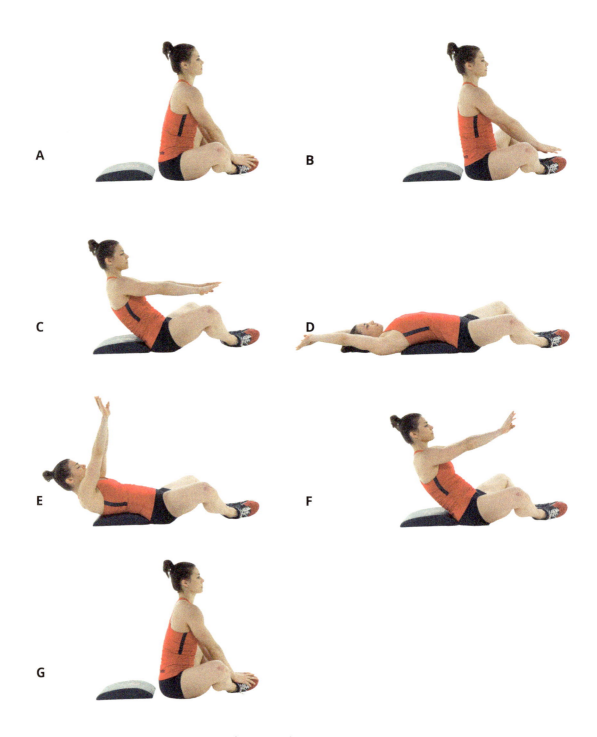

Figure 8. AbMat Sit-up.

all the way to the cervical, finishing with a rhomboid pull back at the top. The initial movement comes out of a powerful, dynamic glute-hamstring movement that extends the hip. Then the back extends sequentially along the spine from "south to north" (Figure 5).

This movement does a lot for a coach. It heightens a neurological awareness. It allows me to introduce some essential vernacular to the client. If we do not have cues that allow me to talk about hip flexion, trunk flexion, hip extension, trunk extension, I am fairly worthless with a client. Very early, get clients to know terms. Be able to call it out and get the response you need.

This movement demonstrates tremendous control. There is hip flexion, hip extension, trunk flexion and trunk extension in a combo "snake" move. Using those muscles is essential for midline stabilization and working the posterior.

The fourth movement on the GHD is a sit-up but involves no trunk flexion. For the GHD sit-up, the pad is set so that the pelvis is free, and the athlete descends back to touch the ground and then comes back to seated. More than a few exercise physiologists and certified trainers have observed that this movement is pure hip flexion and consequently asserted "there's no abs in that."

But what the abs are doing in this exercise is midline stabilization.

Before having clients perform the GHD sit-up, ensure they have demonstrated capacity in the hip extension, back extension, and hip-and-back extension. Even still, their first GHD sit-ups should be performed in a shortened range of motion, with the trainer spotting behind them (Figure 6). That might be it for the first dose. Once they come back and you can determine the effect from that dose, increase the range of motion and volume as their capacity allows.

To perform a GHD sit-up, there is some leg flexion in the descent. Then, the leg extends dramatically and pulls the athlete to seated (Figure 7). Conversely, if the athlete does not extend the leg to come to seated, the primary movers are the hip flexors, but specifically the psoas.

The psoas comes off the femur, runs through the pelvis (without attachment) and attaches to the lumbar spine. The hip flexors also include a very powerful complement to the psoas: the rectus femoris, which is the dominant piece of the quadriceps. The rectus femoris does not attach to the lumbar spine, but it attaches to the pelvis. This attachment to the pelvis is a point of enormous mechanical advantage and leverage. And to fully engage that, the leg must extend dramatically. The leg cannot sharply extend without working rectus femoris—a leg extensor and a hip flexor.

The force with which an athlete comes up is amazing. Rather than being pulled from the psoas alone, which is a fairly dysfunctional kind of pull, the athlete uses the full complement of hip-flexor musculature. Any time you are using a fraction of the primary movers responsible for that articulation, it is not natural, not functional, and contrary to nature. Not extending the leg can also be a little irritating to the low back due to this shearing force on the lumbar spine. Performed correctly, the movement is not irritating to the low back. Straightening that leg enables profound musculature to lift from the pelvis.

There are people who have this irritation in the spine from a shear force. If you can teach them to extend the legs to work the full complement of hip flexors, we will move the margins where this irritation occurs from 3 reps to 4 reps to 10 reps and so on. That is rehabilitation. That is neuromuscular re-education.

There is an adjunct movement to GHD sit-up in which the athlete is dynamic in the trunk and static in the hip. It is the AbMat sit-up, where we deliberately take the hip flexors out of the equation and work the torso dynamically. The hip flexors are working statically or possibly to no significant degree.

To do this, the hip flexors need to be removed from the line of action. The fat part of the AbMat goes toward the glutes, and the athlete puts the bottom of his or her soles together with the knees butterflied. This positioning makes the hip flexors tangential to the line of action; i.e., they cannot do any productive work. This is done deliberately. Then the athlete slowly and under control comes to seated by contracting the abdominals. This is a very dynamic bit of trunk flexion and the hip flexors are removed (Figure 8).

As the athlete fails, adduct and extend the legs to some degree. This creates more purchase for the hip flexors and brings them into the line of action. This allows the athlete to modulate the assistance and keep each rep focused on the midsection.

If reps are performed slowly and deliberately, most athletes will fail a sit-up without an AbMat. The failure is not necessarily a neuromuscular failure. It is not necessarily a weakness or deficiency. The truth is the movement is defective minus the AbMat.

Without an AbMat, the athlete has a solid point of contact below the upper back. To move, I need to act off of something immovable. When the athlete gets full contraction of the rectus, the lower back actually goes flat. This is not enough to bring him up to seated. When this space between the low back and the floor is filled with something to act against (like the AbMat), the athlete can curl to seated.

There is a very short range of motion available in lumbar flexion to protect the spine. The beauty of the spine is that each piece moves a very short range of motion in all directions, and in total they get some pretty cool dynamics. But that lumbar region is fairly inflexible, and all that range of motion that is available moves one from spinally extended through to neutral. There is no more shortening or flexion to it; it is not enough to sit up.

Without the AbMat, the sit-up is a biphasic movement. While I have solid contact, I use upper rectus and create enough momentum to throw the load to the hip flexors, where I have more connection. This means that the full rectus has little stimulus—it is pulling me from spinally extended through to neutral, but absent of any load. The upper rectus is worked where there is a fulcrum, so the back flattens, but it is the hip flexors that pull me to seated. There is no amount of sit-ups you can do on the ground that is ever going to work you from pubic bone to about 3 or 4 inches above the belly button. The AbMat moves the athlete from spinally extended through to neutral in the lumbar spine against a load.

How big would your bench press get if you only pushed air? You would get as strong as your abs will with a ground-based sit-up. With or without the pad, there is the same contraction and range of motion in the midsection. Without the pad, the fibers shortened but there was no load and no real work completed. With the pad, they got the same motion but under a load, and it produced fruitful work.

The two sit-ups, GHD and AbMat, complement each other beautifully. One is dynamic in the hips and static in the trunk; the other is dynamic in the trunk and static in the hip. In conjunction with the L-sit (static in the trunk and hip), they develop a formidable capacity in the midline. ∎

WHERE DO I GO FROM HERE?

When an individual fully participates in the Level 1 Certificate Course and passes the Level 1 test, he or she earns the designation CrossFit Level 1 Trainer (CF-L1). This credential can be used in a resume or biography and is valid for five years from the date of course completion. To maintain the credential, trainers must retake the course every five years (or sooner) or pursue higher-level CrossFit credentials.

The Level 1 Course is an effective, broad survey of CrossFit's foundational methodology and movements, and earning the Level 1 Certificate should be considered the first step for training others. The purpose of this article is to provide guidance for additional professional development of new CrossFit trainers. The article is divided into three sections:

1) How to Be an Effective Trainer.
2) How to Develop as a Trainer.
3) How to Train Others While Gaining Experience.

The term "virtuosity"—doing the common uncommonly well—can be used to describe the mastery of movement technique that CrossFit athletes seek to achieve. Chasing virtuosity can also describe the path to coaching mastery. Master coaches display an unmatched capacity to improve others' fitness. True mastery demands a lifetime commitment to improvement of craft; those looking for mastery never consider their development complete.

HOW TO BE AN EFFECTIVE TRAINER

An effective trainer must have capacity in six different abilities:

- Teaching.
- Seeing.
- Correcting.
- Group and/or gym management.
- Presence and attitude.
- Demonstration.

This list can be viewed as similar in principle to the list of 10 general physical skills for fitness outlined in "What is Fitness? (Part 1)." Athletes with capacity in each of the 10 skills are considered fitter than athletes who demonstrate excessive capacity in any one skill to a detriment of capacity in the others. Similarly, effective trainers demonstrate capacity in each of the six abilities listed above, not just one or two. The more effective the trainer, the greater his or her capacity in each ability. These six areas are the focus of study and practical application at the Level 2 Certificate Course.

> 1. *Teaching—The ability to effectively articulate and teach the mechanics of each movement. This includes the ability to focus on major points*

of performance before more subtle or nuanced ones and the ability to change instruction based on the athlete's needs and capacity.

A trainer's ability to teach others reflects his or her knowledge as well as the ability to effectively communicate that knowledge. To communicate knowledge to others, a coach must understand what defines proper mechanics and what causes bad or inefficient movement. This requires continual study, and one's teaching will improve with greater understanding in all fields that intersect with fitness.

An effective teacher also has a unique ability to relate to every student, regardless of his or her background and ability. This requires the teacher to distill a large body of knowledge to a single point or a few salient points specific to the current need of the athlete and the movement being taught. An effective teacher also takes ownership for recognizing when communication between the teacher and athlete breaks down. Generally, the more forms of communication a teacher employs (verbal, visual, tactile, use of different examples/ analogies, etc.), the more likely the athlete will find success in training.

> 2. *Seeing—The ability to discern good from poor movement mechanics and to identify both gross and subtle faults whether the athlete is in motion or static.*

An effective trainer demonstrates the ability to see movement and determine whether the mechanics are sound or unsound. This ability first requires knowledge of when to observe and evaluate very specific aspects of the athlete's movement (e.g., trunk-to-femur relationship for hip extension, center of pressure on feet for posterior-chain engagement). It also requires knowledge of the differences between good and poor positions. An effective trainer can see faults both when the athlete is moving (e.g., hip extension) and not moving (e.g., the receiving position of a clean). Newer coaches tend to have the greatest difficulty spotting movement faults while athletes are moving.

> 3. *Correcting—The ability to facilitate better mechanics for an athlete using visual, verbal, and/or tactile cues. This includes the ability to triage (prioritize) faults in order of importance, which includes an understanding of how multiple faults are related.*

Once a trainer can teach the movements and see faults, he or she is then able to correct the athlete. Effective correction makes an athlete's mechanics better. Correcting hinges on the trainer's ability to:
- Use successful cues.
- Know multiple corrections for each fault.
- Triage faulty movement.
- Balance critique with praise.

Any cue that results in improved movement mechanics is successful and therefore a "good" cue. There are no specific formulas, formats or rules to follow for cues, and their value is based on the result.

However, short, specific and actionable cues – "push the hips back" – tend to result in a greater success rate. A trainer needs multiple strategies for each fault because different clients often respond to the same cue in a different manner.

When multiple faults occur at once, a trainer is best served by attacking them one at a time in order of importance (i.e., triaging). The ordering is based on the severity of the deviation from ideal and the athlete's capacity relative to the task; no single ordering of faults can be used across all athletes and movements. Throughout the cueing process, a trainer needs to celebrate small changes or even just celebrate hard work to build rapport and acknowledge a client's effort even when those efforts are not immediately successful.

Newer trainers tend to be lacking in their ability to see and correct movement. When coaching others, trainers need to focus on movement. Good coaches relentlessly watch movement with a critical eye. Good coaches are constantly asking the following questions: How could an individual be more efficient and safe? What cues would result in a better position? How can cues be delivered to produce the best response from the athlete? Good coaches produce noticeable changes in their athletes' movement. To develop this critical eye, coaches can work with great trainers, film themselves or other athletes, or film classes.

> 4. *Group Management—The ability to organize and manage, both at a micro level (within each class) and at the macro gym level. This includes managing time well; organization of the space, equipment, and participants for optimal flow and experience; planning ahead; etc.*

Group management speaks to the trainer's ability to reduce the logistical set-up and preparation time during a class to maximize the amount of teaching and movement time. This means the trainer plans the instruction ahead of time (see "Running a CrossFit Class" article) and perhaps pre-arranges the equipment and/or weights to avoid excessive talking at the expense of moving.

Practice time in every class is necessary for both the trainer and client. Practice time gives the trainer time to observe and cue movement mechanics, and it gives the client time to work on movement with improved form. Every student should feel he or she received personal coaching within the group atmosphere. Regardless of each athlete's experience, trainers should make an honest assessment of the time and attention given to each client after each training session. The goal is to maximize a trainer's effectiveness and reach.

5. *Presence and Attitude—The ability to create a positive and engaging learning environment. The trainer shows empathy for athletes and creates rapport.*

Although presence and attitude are more intangible than the other criteria, clients immediately feel their absence. "Positive" should not be interpreted as fake or forced. A trainer should be authentic, with a goal of creating a positive training experience for clients. A positive learning environment might take many different forms, and an effective trainer recognizes each person has different needs and goals. It is the trainer's responsibility to determine how to relate to and motivate each individual in order to help him or her reach stated goals. An effective trainer demonstrates interpersonal skills by interacting and communicating clearly with each client individually.

Care, empathy, and a passion for service are traits commonly displayed by trainers with positive presence and attitude. Effective trainers care about improving the quality of their clients' lives. Clients perceive this care more quickly than they perceive a trainer's ability to explain mechanics, anatomy or nutrition.

6. *Demonstration—The ability to provide athletes with an accurate visual example of the movement at hand. Demonstration also includes the concept of leading by example: A trainer should follow his or her own advice and be an inspiration to clients.*

A trainer must be able to provide a visual demonstration of the movement. Demonstration is a useful teaching tool to show safe and efficient movement and range-of-motion standards. It requires a strong awareness of one's own movement mechanics. It is acceptable to use others for this purpose in cases of physical limitations. A trainer with a good eye should have no problem quickly finding someone for this purpose.

Demonstration extends beyond moving well in a single class; demonstration also means a trainer leads by example, adhering to the same range-of-motion standards as his or her clients, following his or her own programming or nutrition advice, or putting forth the positive and supportive attitude he or she wants to see in clients.

While understanding the necessity of these six qualities is simple, the challenge is simultaneously demonstrating them in a dynamic environment such as group coaching. A commitment to improving each area is the hallmark of a successful trainer, regardless of the trainer's current level of proficiency. Just as the athlete must refine and improve movement mechanics, a trainer must refine coaching skills across a career to become great. Doing so develops virtuosity in coaching.

There is a compelling tendency among novices developing any skill or art, whether learning to play the violin, write poetry, or compete in gymnastics, to quickly move past the fundamentals and on to more elaborate, more sophisticated movements, skills, or techniques. This compulsion is the novice's curse - the rush to originality and risk."

–COACH GLASSMAN

HOW TO DEVELOP AS A TRAINER

To keep up with athletes' progress, a coach must continue to refine and develop his or her knowledge. If a trainer's clients are not testing the limits of his or her knowledge, the trainer is not doing a good enough job with them. An expert coach is eager and proud to have a student exceed his or her abilities but seeks to delay it by staying ahead of the athlete's needs rather than by retarding the athlete's growth. Coaches should focus on development in both academic and practical environments.

Here are some suggestions for how trainers can develop:

1) First and foremost, teach to learn. It is only through experience that a trainer will learn and gain competency. It is imperative to work with people in a dynamic environment, even if they are friends or family in the beginning. Understanding biochemistry, anatomy and teaching methodologies is important and supportive of this endeavor, but it is not enough to allow a trainer to apply knowledge in real time.

2) Watch more experienced coaches—regardless of their specific discipline. Watch what they watch and when they watch for it. Listen to their cues. The best coaches often need very few words to produce noticeable improvement in mechanics. Also watch their rapport with clients. What draws clients to them?

3) Film yourself coaching others. This can also help with your ability to see and correct movement faults as you have the luxury of slowing down the footage. Be critical of yourself and use the six criteria detailed above to assess strengths and areas for improvement.

4) Attend a Level 2 Certificate Course (L2). The L2 allows trainers to work on their coaching (specifically seeing and correcting movement) in the presence of their peers. Where the Level 1 Course is important for understanding the conceptual framework of CrossFit, the goal of the L2 is to improve one's coaching skill set. The course is designed to give trainers practical feedback based on the six qualities of an effective trainer. It also provides practical drills for trainers to improve specific coaching areas.

5) Attend additional courses. Specialty teaching methods might differ from the general information provided in the Level 1 Course. Instead of focusing on the differences in methods, focus on understanding the concepts of how and why differing methodologies are appropriate for different applications.

CrossFit also offers online courses, such as Scaling and Spot the Flaw. Under its Certification branch, CrossFit offers courses on topics such as anatomy and physiology and best business practices. Those pursing advanced credentials in CrossFit may use these courses for required continuing-education credits, but the courses are open to anyone.

6) Read and study everything related to training, movement and health.

7) Study and follow CrossFit.com. The archives (since 2001) contain years of original CrossFit programming. It is a great resource for learning and experimenting with workouts. We challenge all trainers to follow CrossFit.com programming for at least six months to understand well-varied and challenging CrossFit programming. It provides a good model for the type of workouts, the variance and the volume (i.e., one workout a day) required for long-term results. It will also provide experience on how to scale appropriately, as only the most advanced athletes can complete all CrossFit.com workouts as prescribed (Rx'd).

8) Pursue higher credentials, such as CrossFit Level 2 Trainer, Certified CrossFit Trainer (Level 3) and Certified CrossFit Coach (Level 4). More information about the Level 2 credential can be found on CrossFit.com/certificate-courses, and more information about the certifications can be found on CrossFit.com/certifications. The CrossFit Level 4 Coach credential is the preeminent trainer designation offered by CrossFit. This evaluation provides distinction for expert coaches within the community.

HOW TO TRAIN OTHERS WHILE GAINING EXPERTISE

Expert training comes from years of experience and study long after the completion of the Level 1 Certificate Course. However, a novice or less experienced person can still train others. Three important principles should guide trainers at all levels:

- Master the fundamentals.
- Limit the scope.
- Pursue excellence.

Master the Fundamentals

New athletes are most successful when adhering to the charter of mechanics, consistency and then intensity. Coaches often manage the time frame in which clients reach high levels of intensity. A trainer should not be fooled into thinking new clients need overly complex movements and high-volume workouts to be "sold" on his or her services. Coach Glassman wrote specifically about this in the 2005 article "Fundamentals, Virtuosity, and Mastery: An Open Letter to CrossFit Trainers." Trainers need to take time teaching clients proper mechanics and ensuring they move correctly before high levels of intensity are applied. Insist on consistently safe and correct mechanics, then very gradually increase load and volume—watching closely for movement faults. Not only does this decrease the risk for injury, but it also sets athletes up for greater success in the long term: Efficient and sound mechanics allow ever-increasing speeds and loads. These guidelines enable trainers to learn and gain experience while safeguarding the health and well-being of people in their care.

Applying intensity at either end of the spectrum–too much too soon or too little/none at all–blunts the overall benefit from the program. Pushing one's limits drives new adaptation, and this cannot happen without intensity. On the other hand, pushing too hard too soon can result in long-term inefficiencies or injury. When the trainer is in doubt, it is better to err on the side of caution and progress slowly. Even at low intensity, many participants see benefits simply from performing varied functional movements, and it will become clear over time when intensity can be added.

Limit the Scope

Many CrossFit affiliates follow a group-class model, which can be difficult for a novice coach. The demands of teaching and class management often take the attention away from seeing and correcting movement. New trainers are encouraged to coach friends and family in individual or small group sessions (two or three athletes) to perfect their ability to improve mechanics before taking on large group classes. Another option is to assist a head coach for classes and small-group training. The new trainer can improve his or her ability to discern poor movement and cue good movement, while the head trainer addresses the other logistics. New trainers should seek out internships or assistant roles at local affiliates to gain this experience. A trainer needs to increase the size of classes gradually to continually deliver quality training, as Coach Glassman articulated in 2006 in "Scaling Professional Training":

> "To run group classes without compromising our hallmark laser focus and commitment to the athlete, the trainer has to learn to give each member of the group the impression that he is getting all the attention that he could get in one-on-one training, and that requires tremendous training skill. We've seen this skill fully and adequately developed by only one path–gradually migrating from one-on-one to group sessions. ... There's no way a new trainer can walk into this environment and do well."

Beyond the demands of running one quality class is the demand of delivering that quality training for multiple sessions a day. As Coach Glassman wrote when training in Santa Cruz, California: "Five appointments per day is about all we could handle without an unacceptable drop in energy, focus, and, consequently, professional standards."

Limiting the scope also means trainers should have the clarity and self-awareness to admit when they do not know something. Whether it is a question regarding anatomy in the squat, why someone has back pain or why excess sugar can compromise health, it is not wise to try to make up information when an issue is beyond the current level of knowledge or scope of practice. Working only within the limits of one's knowledge will help protect the safety of clients and build credibility. A trainer cannot be expected to know all things related to health and fitness. Develop and foster a community of other professionals clients can be referred to with confidence when necessary. Seek to learn the answers to any questions, and in the case of any medical condition, the trainer should always refer the client to a physician.

Pursue Excellence

To be a successful trainer (or affiliate), CrossFit's recommended "business model" is the relentless and continual pursuit of excellence. Pursuing excellence was the guiding tenet from the early days of the original CrossFit gym in Santa Cruz, and the concept continues to guide larger decisions related to CrossFit.com and the Level 1 Certificate Course, for example. The overarching purpose is to bring more quality training to more people. Rather than devising a business model in the pursuit of money, devise one that is focused on making the training (and, by extension, the clients) better. The most effective business plan comes from achieving excellence and letting the market bring the money to you.

To pursue excellence, ask the question, "What would make the training or the affiliate better?" An analysis of pros and cons can muddle every decision, and most issues can be decided by a simple question: "Will it improve the quality of the programming or the training experience?" If the answer is "Yes!" you are most likely pursuing excellence.

CROSSFIT COMMUNITY AND REPRESENTATION

The Level 1 Certificate Course is a great way to formalize one's involvement in the CrossFit community. It provides the conceptual framework of the program. It also serves to transmit the community's ethos: a sense of camaraderie and support among like-minded individuals who are humble, hard-working and committed to service.

Along with our affiliates, those who become Level 1 Trainers are the community's most important ambassadors. The CF-L1 credential is the first step toward affiliation; more information on that process can be found on CrossFit.com. The global community is more than 13,000 affiliates strong. Whether working at an existing affiliate or opening a new affiliate, each CrossFit trainer can positively influence lives every day. It is the daily effort of performing constantly varied functional movements at high intensity coupled with a diet of meat and vegetables, nuts and seeds, some fruit, little starch and no sugar that can reverse the tide of chronic disease. It can empower people to achieve feats they never thought possible, even outside the gym. It can dramatically improve people's quality of life, as well as provide a social and supportive network. One of the best times to witness the power of the community is during the CrossFit Games Open, when more than 380,000 people worldwide come together to test their fitness and–more importantly–push each other to be better than yesterday.

The greater CrossFit community is changing mainstream beliefs about fitness, nutrition and physique. While the goal of CrossFit, Inc. has always been to favorably affect more people with CrossFit training, it is the worldwide community that drives these changes. CrossFit wants its trainers to be a vibrant and engaged addition to the community. Feedback is always welcomed at coursefeedback@crossfit.com; your comments ensure that CrossFit, Inc. best supports its aims.

CrossFit hopes that its trainers care about and protect the community as they would care about and protect anything they value and respect. Thousands of CrossFit trainers have used the Level 1 Certificate Course as a springboard to their coaching careers. New trainers should use the material learned from the Level 1 Course and this guide and slowly apply it to others, incrementally increasing their scope over time. This continued development will eventually lead to coaching virtuosity. ∎

RESPONSIBLE TRAINING

Being an expert coach is about improving fitness and safeguarding the health of one's clients. Keeping clients safe includes knowing the movement points of performance and being able to identify and correct violations. However, client safety also includes multiple logistical factors, such as programming, specific needs for special populations, equipment layout and accurate representation of one's credentials. This article is meant to prime new Level 1 Trainers to responsibly train others while gaining expertise.

MITIGATE CLIENTS' RISK OF RHABDOMYOLYSIS

Rhabdomyolysis, while rare, can develop from high-intensity or high-volume exercise, including CrossFit or any other process that damages muscle cells. Rhabdomyolysis (often simply referred to as "rhabdo") is a medical condition that might arise from breakdown of muscle tissue and release of the muscle cells' contents into the bloodstream. This process can damage the kidneys and can lead to renal failure or death in rare cases. Rhabdo is diagnosed when a patient with an appropriate history has an elevated level of creatine kinase, also known as CK or CPK. CPK is easier to measure in the blood than myoglobin and is generally used as a marker for rhabdo, even though it is the myoglobin that does the damage.

Treatment consists of generous amounts of intravenous (IV) fluids to dilute and flush the myoglobin through the kidneys. In the worst cases, patients might need dialysis while the kidneys recover. Death, though rare, can result when kidney failure causes imbalances in the usual electrolytes, which can cause cardiac arrhythmias. Most patients make a complete recovery after being rehydrated with IV fluids over anywhere from several hours to a week or so, depending on the severity.

There are a few ways a CrossFit trainer can protect athletes from rhabdomyolysis:
- Follow the charter of mechanics, consistency, intensity.
- Know the movements that have a higher rate of rhabdomyolysis incidence (those that prolong the eccentric contraction), and be mindful of the total volume that is programmed with these exercises.
- Scale workouts for clients appropriately.
- Avoid progressive scaling.
- Educate clients on the symptoms of rhabdomyolysis and when it is appropriate to seek medical attention.

Following the mechanics-consistency-intensity charter best prepares the athlete for long-term success, but it is also a way to mitigate the potential of developing rhabdomyolysis (and other injuries). Slow and gradual increases in intensity and volume allow the body to acclimate to high-intensity and higher-volume exercise. Even athletes who quickly demonstrate sound mechanics still need a gradual increase in intensity and volume. When working with new athletes, trainers should focus on using modest loads, reducing volume and coaching the athlete on technique. At affiliates where there are "elements" or "on-ramp" classes that last a couple of weeks, athletes should still be heavily scaled beyond this introductory period to ensure adequate time to acclimate to CrossFit training. If there are no separate classes for beginners, treat the workouts as technique sessions for newer athletes–focus on their mechanics rather than speed or load. There is no set protocol for how quickly to increase intensity, but it is wise to err on the side of caution and work toward long-term fitness. Multiple months at scaled loads and volumes are well within a normal timeframe for even the best athletes, with gradual increases in intensity implemented after that. Trainers need to frequently check in with athletes to determine how the previous dose of exercise affected them. Although intensity is a significant part of CrossFit, each athlete has his or her entire life to continue to improve fitness and tolerance for intensity.

The second way to mitigate the risk of rhabdomyolysis is to know the movements associated with a higher rate of incidence. Beginner athletes should keep "negatives" (movements which prolong the eccentric phase) to a minimum. Although negatives can be an effective way to increase strength, they should not be used in high volumes with beginners. Athletes may increase the volume of negatives gradually over time.

While the eccentric phase of movements cannot and should not be avoided, there are movements in which people are more likely to prolong the eccentric phase. In CrossFit, these tend to be jumping pull-ups and full-range-of-motion glute-ham developer (GHD) sit-ups. In the jumping pull-up, the athlete should not prolong the descent but should instead immediately drop to an extended-arm position once the chin has cleared the bar, absorbing the impact with the legs. Similarly, in the full-range-of-motion GHD sit-up, newer athletes should use fewer repetitions and potentially a shortened range of motion until capacity is developed. It is also prudent for trainers to scale the number of repetitions and the range of motion for athletes who do not routinely use GHD sit-ups regardless of their CrossFit experience. There are no exact rules for total volume, but beginners and new CrossFit athletes (and even advanced CrossFit athletes who have not been routinely using the GHD) should start with relatively low repetitions of the partial-range-of-motion GHD sit-up (i.e., to parallel) and gradually increase from there with consistent exposure.

Progressive scaling–the practice of continually adjusting the difficulty of a workout so that an exhausted athlete can keep moving–must be avoided with the beginner or even intermediate athlete. Allow these athletes to stop and take rest as needed to complete the workout. An example: A trainer keeps lowering the load so the athlete does not have to stop completing reps (e.g., 135-lb. barbell for thrusters dropped to 115 to 95 to 65 to 45 across the workout duration). Progressive scaling may be used, but it must be applied very cautiously even with the most advanced of athletes.

It is also wise to educate athletes about the potential risk for rhabdomyolysis, strategies to reduce the risk and the symptoms. This will help them understand the rationale for scaling their workouts, especially when they are zealous to perform a workout "as prescribed" ("Rx'd").

Alcohol and drug use increase the risk of rhabdomyolysis, and athletes should avoid heavy drinking, especially in proximity to training. Certain medications, including statins (cholesterol-lowering agents), increase the risk of rhabdomyolysis.

Symptoms of rhabdomyolysis include severe generalized muscle pain, nausea and vomiting, abdominal cramping, and, in severe cases, dark-red or cola-colored urine. The discoloration of the urine comes from the muscle's myoglobin, which is the same molecule that gives red meat its color. If these symptoms appear following a workout (or at any time with regard to dark-red urine), the athlete should seek medical attention immediately.

The athletes at highest risk seem to be those with a reasonable baseline level of fitness obtained through some non-CrossFit training, those who are returning to CrossFit after a layoff, or even experienced CrossFit athletes who reach volume or intensity significantly outside their established "norm." These athletes have sufficient muscle mass and conditioning to create enough intensity to hurt themselves. Generally, the most deconditioned seem to be at less risk (but not zero). It is suspected they do not have enough muscle mass or the capacity to generate high levels of intensity. This being said, trainers must properly scale and focus on mechanics with every client regardless of current capacity.

MINIMIZE EQUIPMENT- AND SPOTTING-RELATED INJURIES

Beyond following the charter of mechanics, consistency, and intensity, affiliate owners can further minimize risk of injury within their gym. Very real risks exist from equipment condition, use, and arrangement, as well as from improper spotting of athletes during movements.

Equipment condition refers both to installation and day-to-day maintenance. Installation often applies to building pull-up rigs, hanging gymnastics rings, assembling a GHD, among other things. Professional assistance should be used when an owner is inexperienced.

Pull-up-bar rigs and gymnastic rings and associated straps should be designed to bear a load far higher than the expected maximum weight to be supported. These structures need to be tested at maximum loading before regular client use.

Regularly scheduled maintenance of all equipment is paramount. Equipment that places the athlete's feet off the ground or inverts the athlete requires extra time and attention. Support pieces like straps, racks or bars and locking mechanisms need to be kept in working order and checked regularly for routine wear. Some might become compromised during use. Where there is a risk for handles or collars to come apart, dumbbells, kettlebells, and even barbells need to be inspected regularly for integrity. Trainers must repair, replace, and discontinue use of faulty equipment immediately.

Arrangement refers to the layout of equipment and athletes during a class or workout. Each athlete needs enough space to perform the movements, with an additional buffer to account for the errant-moving equipment, missed attempts, and safe passage of coaches or other athletes. Under no circumstances should a trainer permit extra equipment like bars, plates, boxes, etc. to be left lying around the workout area. This equipment might trip athletes or cause a ricochet if other equipment lands on it.

It is also imperative for a trainer to prepare for falls during dynamic movements. It is possible that an athlete might lose his or her grip during a kip (pull-up or muscle-up). Trainers might encourage athletes to wrap their thumbs around any bar in an effort to provide additional feedback to the athlete. This is not foolproof, however, and can sometimes be even less secure, particularly for athletes with small hands. Whatever the hand position chosen, it does not replace the need for the athlete to develop body awareness of when to end the movement if his or her grip is compromised (wrapping thumbs is always recommended for barbell and ring movements to help provide better balance and control, especially in higher-risk scenarios such as a bench press or muscle-up). Boxes and racks should not be beneath, behind or directly in front of these athletes. Adjustable rings should be lowered to the appropriate height. Where assistance boxes are necessary, they are best placed to the side of the working athlete (and not in another athlete's way) to leave a clear path should an athlete leave the apparatus prematurely. A suggestion for trainers trying to manage these risks is to do a "dry run" of the workout before it begins: check the working space for each athlete for each of the proposed movements. This can be as simple as organizing the class to rotate stations on the trainer's call and perform a quick walk-through to check spacing and arrangement. Trainers can then instruct participants to move to the same spot during the workout to ensure safety.

Athletes also need instruction regarding how to bail safely from lifts and how to spot other athletes where appropriate. In most weightlifting movements, the athletes only need to learn how to bail safely. Trainers need to teach athletes this skill and allow them to practice it before any significant load is lifted. Trainers should also ensure enough empty space exists around a working athlete so a missed lift does not have a ricochet effect, as mentioned above. Spotting is not recommended for weightlifting movements, except for a bench press (where it is mandatory) and potentially a back squat (especially where a low-bar position is used). A trainer cannot assume athletes understand how to spot correctly, and again, instruction and practice at lighter loads are necessary.

Experienced trainers or athletes may also provide a spot for gymnastics movements. Trainers or athletes should employ a spot that minimizes risk to both spotter and athlete. Generally, gymnastics movements are spotted at the torso or hips to provide adequate support for the movement, but spotting at the hips or legs can be successful (e.g., handstands). The spotter may be to the rear of the athlete if the risk of getting hit is low (e.g., ring support, GHD sit-up), but often a position beside the athlete is best (e.g., handstand).

Trainers need to be sure equipment is cleaned regularly to reduce the chance of infection, and proper disinfectants and sterilizers, with clean cloths, should be staged near the gym floor to clean blood off bars immediately. A blood-spill clean-up procedure can be found in the CrossFit Journal archives.

MONITORING ATHLETES FOR CONDITIONS THAT NEED MEDICAL ATTENTION

Although a trainer is primarily there to instruct and improve athlete movements, he or she needs to monitor the level of exertion during the workout and ensure athlete health is protected. As CrossFit workouts use relatively high intensity, athletes are working at their physical and psychological tolerances. It is possible for athletes to push too hard, and confounding environmental factors might exacerbate certain situations.

Extreme temperature fluctuations, especially heat, can be problematic. Trainers should be ready in unseasonably hot and humid weather with sufficient water, and they should watch for common signs of overexertion (e.g., dizziness). Hot weather also increases the potential risk for rhabdomyolysis (although some cases have occurred in cold climates), and trainers should encourage athletes to stay hydrated (with the caveat that they should not be excessively hydrated. Current mainstream literature suggests rates of 1.2 L/hour, which are actually too high and can lead to overhydration). In the event of a potential heat stroke following a workout (e.g., athlete demonstrates an altered mental state), a trainer should remove excess clothing from the athlete and then douse him or her with cool water before medical attention arrives.

Weather aside, other conditions might need medical attention. Symptoms such as numbness or chronic pain in joints and muscles should be referred to medical professionals. Medical attention is immediately necessary for any non-responsive athlete.

Trainers can be best prepared for medical emergencies by getting trained in cardio-pulmonary resuscitation (CPR) and the use of an automatic external defibrillator (AED), and by having an AED at the gym. Most states require this by law, and CrossFit trainers and affiliates should ensure they are in compliance with all state laws. CPR/AED credentials often last for one or two years depending on the organization (e.g., Red Cross, American Heart Association), and trainers should keep them current.

HYDRATION

Drink when you are thirsty, do not when you are not.

We advise against rehydration strategies that encourage consumption of fluids to prevent loss of body-weight during activity. Dehydration during physical activity is a normal physiological process, and the thirst mechanism is sufficient in regulating hydration and serum sodium concentration during exercise.

Drinking beyond thirst in an attempt to prevent body-weight loss during exercise offers no benefit to health or performance. It also presents a serious risk of exercise-associated hyponatremia (EAH), a potentially deadly dilution of the body's serum sodium concentration. EAH is caused by overconsumption of fluid and can be viewed as an iatrogenic condition due to the prevailing belief that exercising athletes should drink "as much fluid as tolerable" during training.

"Fluid" that can contribute to EAH includes electrolyte-enhanced sports drinks. Contrary to popular belief, these commercial beverages do not reduce risk of hyponatremia. Because of flavoring and sugar content, these drinks might present greater risk for overconsumption of fluid than water alone, increasing the risk of potentially deadly EAH in athletes.

SPECIAL POPULATIONS
Any potential athlete with a medical condition needs to be cleared by a physician for exercise before a trainer recommends a fitness regimen. A medical-history form can be a useful tool for a trainer to assess any potential issues, although trainers are also encouraged to ask questions regarding medical status and be aware of common medical conditions that need clearance (e.g., diabetes, prescription medications).

Common special populations include pregnant athletes, and a trainer should still request medical clearance and guidelines from the physician once the condition is known. The CrossFit Journal archive contains many resources regarding scaling for pregnant athletes, such as the article "Pregnancy: A Practical Guide for Scaling." A trainer should be especially aware of reducing the risk of potential falls in workouts (e.g., box jumps, rope climbs) and be observant for complaints of calf pain or swelling, which can be signs of more serious issues.

Many athletes have found improved recovery while staying active after surgery. While CrossFit workouts are indeed scalable for these athletes, trainers should seek clearance from the surgeon before restarting a workout regimen with them.

A trainer's scope of practice allows promotion of any individual's desire to participate in exercise and provision of direction; this does not extend to diagnosing or treating any medical condition.

LEGAL USE OF THE "CROSSFIT LEVEL 1 TRAINER" CREDENTIAL
Passing the exam at the Level 1 Certificate Course earns an individual the designation of CrossFit Level 1 Trainer, which can be abbreviated "CF-L1 Trainer." The American National Standards Institute (ANSI), the third party through which the course is accredited, has approved this title.

It is important for CrossFit trainers to:
- Use the correct terminology for the credential.
- Act in accordance with the Level 1 Trainer Certificate License Agreement.

Participants sign this document as part of receiving their test results.

A CrossFit Level 1 Trainer holds the Level 1 Certificate. The Certificate is valid for a period of five years. See the Participant Handbook for details regarding maintaining an active trainer status. CrossFit's public Trainer Directory can be used to verify any individual's credentials. Those who pass the exam should not use the term "certified." While the distinction in terminology appears minor, the use of "Level 1 Certified" is a misrepresentation of the credential and is not endorsed by CrossFit. A "Certificate Course," such as the Level 1 Certificate Course, is a course with learning objectives and a test that is tied to those specific objectives. It includes both an educational or "training" component as well as a test to determine if the participant has learned the course material. A "certification," such as the Certified CrossFit Trainer or Certified CrossFit Coach credential, is only a test with no educational component. Certifications are designed to assess competency across an entire profession. Preparation work for the certifications is done on the applicant's own time and under his or her own guidance. In layman's terms, and in the case of the CrossFit credentials, a certification generally demonstrates a greater scope of professional competency versus a certificate.

The CrossFit Level 1 Trainer credential may be used next to one's name similar to other educational credentials (e.g., M.S., R.N., D.C.). It may be used on a website with a biography or on a business card. It does not allow use of the name "CrossFit" to market services (e.g., personal CrossFit training, CrossFit classes). To market services, a trainer must first apply to run a CrossFit affiliate.

During the Level 1 Course, participants were exposed to a large amount of knowledge. Much of it can be found elsewhere free to the public and is commonly known to or accepted by the fitness industry in some form. However, this knowledge is not found so organized and packaged outside the Level 1 Course. This defines the CrossFit method. An individual can use the CrossFit method to train himself or herself and friends and family without charge. However, to use the CrossFit name or logo (i.e., the CrossFit brand) to market services, a Level 1 Trainer must affiliate. An individual is not permitted to advertise, market, promote or solicit, in business or service, without licensing the CrossFit name. Licensing the CrossFit name is called "affiliation." More information regarding affiliation can be found on CrossFit.com.

The risk-to-benefit ratio for CrossFit participants is very low; however, it is also the trainer's responsibility to maintain the low risk for his or her clients. The guidance presented here should serve as a resource for new CrossFit trainers to keep clients safe in the gym. ▪

FUNDAMENTALS, VIRTUOSITY AND MASTERY:
AN OPEN LETTER TO CROSSFIT TRAINERS

Originally published in August 2005.

In gymnastics, completing a routine without error will not get you a perfect score, the 10.0—only a 9.7. To get the last three tenths of a point, you must demonstrate "risk, originality, and virtuosity" as well as make no mistakes in execution of the routine.

Risk is simply executing a movement that is likely to be missed or botched; originality is a movement or combination of movements unique to the athlete—a move or sequence not seen before. Understandably, novice gymnasts love to demonstrate risk and originality, for both are dramatic, fun, and awe inspiring—especially among the athletes themselves, although audiences are less likely to be aware when either is demonstrated.

Virtuosity, though, is a different beast altogether. Virtuosity is defined in gymnastics as "performing the common uncommonly well." Unlike risk and originality, virtuosity is elusive, supremely elusive. It is, however, readily recognized by the audience as well as coaches and athletes. But more importantly, more to my point, virtuosity is more than the requirement for that last tenth of a point; it is always the mark of true mastery (and of genius and beauty).

There is a compelling tendency among novices developing any skill or art, whether learning to play the violin, write poetry, or compete in gymnastics, to quickly move past the fundamentals and on to more elaborate, more sophisticated movements, skills, or techniques. This compulsion is the novice's curse–the rush to originality and risk.

The novice's curse is manifested as excessive adornment, silly creativity, weak fundamentals and, ultimately, marked lack of virtuosity and delayed mastery. If you have ever had the opportunity to be taught by the very best in any field you have likely been surprised at how simple, how fundamental, how basic the instruction was. The novice's curse afflicts learner and teacher alike. Physical training is no different.

What will inevitably doom a physical training program and dilute a coach's efficacy is a lack of commitment to fundamentals. We see this increasingly in both programming and supervising execution. Rarely now do we see prescribed the short, intense couplets or triplets that epitomize CrossFit programming. Rarely do trainers really nitpick the mechanics of fundamental movements.

I understand how this occurs. It is natural to want to teach people advanced and fancy movements. The urge to quickly move away from the basics and toward advanced movements arises out of the natural desire to entertain your client and impress him with your skills and knowledge. But make no mistake: it is a sucker's move. Teaching a snatch where there is not yet an overhead squat, teaching an overhead squat where there is not yet an air squat, is a colossal mistake. This rush to advancement increases the chance of injury, delays advancement and progress, and blunts the client's rate of return on his efforts. In short, it retards his fitness.

If you insist on basics, really insist on them, your clients will immediately recognize that you are a master trainer. They will not be bored; they will be awed. I promise this. They will quickly come to recognize the potency of fundamentals. They will also advance in every measurable way past those not blessed to have a teacher so grounded and committed to basics.

Training will improve, clients will advance faster, and you will appear more experienced and professional and garner more respect if you simply recommit to the basics.

There is plenty of time within an hour session to warm up, practice a basic movement or skill or pursue a new personal record (PR) or max lift, discuss and critique the athletes' efforts, and then pound out a tight little couplet or triplet utilizing these skills or just play. Play is important. Tire flipping, basketball, relay races, tag, Hoover-ball, and the like are essential to good programming, but they are seasoning–like salt, pepper, and oregano. They are not main courses.

CrossFit trainers have the tools to be the best trainers on Earth. I really believe that. But good enough never is, and we want that last tenth of a point, the whole 10.0. We want virtuosity! ▪

PROFESSIONAL TRAINING

Originally published in January 2006.

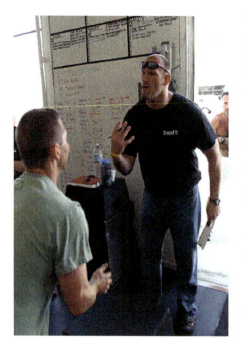

I am a fitness trainer. My practice is more than just a job; it is my passion. My clients are my top priority and their successes are my life's work–I am a professional.

On the surface, my job is to shepherd my athletes (I view all my clients as athletes regardless of their age or ability) toward physical prowess, but I recognize a purpose to my efforts and an impact on my athletes that transcends the physical. I view training as a physical metaphor for habits and attitudes that foster success in all arenas. I stress that point to all who train with me, and I know I have been successful only after they bring back concrete examples.

> "If a trainer's clients are not testing the limits of his knowledge, he is not doing a good enough job with them."
>
> –COACH GLASSMAN

The lessons learned through physical training are unavoidable. The character traits required and developed through physical training are universally applicable to all endeavors. Perseverance, industry, sacrifice, self-control, integrity, honesty, and commitment are best and easiest learned in the gym. Even clients who have found spectacular success in business, sport, war, or love find their most important values buttressed, refined, and nourished in rigorous training.

Being a professional, I believe that my competency is solely determined by my efficacy. My methods must be second to none. Accordingly, fitness trends and fashions are distractions, not attractions. To the extent that my methods are often unconventional, unaccepted, or unique, they reflect the margins by which I dominate my industry, and I take those margins to the bank. A trainer who lusts for popular approval is chasing mediocrity or worse.

Committed to unrivaled efficacy, I have often had to develop new tools and methods. This cannot be done without study and experimentation; consequently, a lot of my work is done not in the gym but in books and scientific literature and in communication with other trainers and coaches.

My competency is determined by my efficacy, which is ultimately determined by my athletes' performance–performance that must be measured. Competition, testing, and recordkeeping let me know the difference between merely looking or feeling good and actually being good at what I do.

My commitment to my athletes is clearly expressed and perceived in our first meeting. I am all theirs. They are the object of my focus and the focus of my conversation. They come back not because of my physical capacity but because they believe in my capacity to develop theirs. World-class athletes rarely make world-class trainers.

I understand that the modern and near-universal trend of skill-less and low-skill programming delivers inferior results and makes cheerleaders of trainers. I will have none of it. I have to understand the mechanics, cues, and techniques of complex movements and to be able to teach them to others. I bring a skill set to my training that scares off most trainers.

Keeping up with my athletes' progress demands that I continue to refine and advance my understanding of advanced skills. If a trainer's clients are not testing the limits of his knowledge, he is not doing a good enough job with them. The master trainer is eager and proud to have a student exceed his abilities but seeks to delay it by staying ahead of the athlete's needs rather than by retarding the athlete's growth.

Because I want my clients' training experience to transcend the physical realm, I am obligated to understand their jobs, hobbies, families, and goals. Motivating clients to transcend fitness requires that I be involved in their lives. This is not going to happen without my being both interested in them and interesting to them.

Being a voracious reader of books, newspapers, and magazines, I have no shortage of conversation, ideas, and knowledge to share, and so you will find me at my clients' parties, weddings, and family gatherings. Indeed, I am a personal friend to nearly every one of my clients. This is extremely gratifying work and often emotionally charged, but that is all right because I am an integral part of my athletes' lives, and life is full of laughter, tears, and hope.

Our friendship, the fun we have, and the frequency of our contact, coupled with the scope of fitness's impact and the technical merits of my training, contribute to a professional relationship with my clients that they value uniquely.

In appreciation, they do all my marketing. I do not advertise, promote, or market. I train very, very well. The more clients I get, the more clients they bring. I do not have time for promotion; I am too busy training. ∎

SCALING PROFESSIONAL TRAINING

Originally published in January 2006.

The standards expressed in "Professional Training"—unyielding commitment to client and efficacy–have guided everything that we have done. More than just the backbone of CrossFit's strength and successes, it has been, we believe, the primary reason for our success.

Using this template, we built a practice that kept us both busy from roughly 5 to 10 a.m. Monday through Saturday. That schedule produced a low-six-figure income, which is really amazing given that we got to work together, with our friends, having a positive impact on people's lives, and keep afternoons free for family, recreation, and study.

The trainers who are running group classes without growing into them are typically not working to the professional training standards that we have described."

–COACH GLASSMAN

Training with the attention and commitment that we bring to our practice, though fun and immensely rewarding, is also draining, and five appointments per day is about all we could handle without an unacceptable drop in energy, focus, and, consequently, professional standards.

Eventually, the demand for our training exceeded the time we were professionally able or willing to allot. In an effort to accommodate more athletes, we began to hold group classes.

We had used group classes to train some of our athletic teams, and everyone loved them, trainers and athletes alike. The social dynamic of group classes is extremely powerful. Run correctly, they motivate an athletic output that is only rarely matched in one-on-one training. The competition and camaraderie of the group classes motivated our line "men will die for points" and the recognition that CrossFit is "the sport of fitness."

Group classes also dramatically increase training revenues!

There are, however, two drawbacks to group classes. The first is space–more athletes require more space to train, but, fortunately, the space required to train 10 people is not 10 times that required for one, and space adequate for one athlete can serve three or four athletes well.

The second drawback is that the reduced trainer-to-trainee ratio can dilute the professional training standards that we have embraced. This natural dilution can, however, be compensated for by the trainer's development of a skill set that is only very rarely found.

To run group classes without compromising our hallmark laser focus and commitment to the athlete, the trainer has to learn to give each member of the group the impression that he is getting all the attention that he could get in one-on-one training, and that requires tremendous training skill.

We have seen this skill fully and adequately developed by only one path: gradually migrating from one-on-one to group sessions. The trainers who are running group classes without growing into them are typically not working to the professional training standards that we have described. They also seem to have an inordinate difficulty filling their classes.

This is exactly how we built our group classes. After working for years at the limit of our one-on-one capacity, we started accepting new clients by doubling them up with other one-on-one clients to form one-on-two appointments.

We introduced the shift to group classes by telling the existing one-on-one clients that we had good news for them: "Your training rate is going to go down and we're going to introduce you to a new friend." Where there was resistance to sharing the time we asked for a trial period. It went swimmingly well.

We structured payment so that a client who was paying, say, $75 per session would now be paying only $50. This drives the trainer's hourly revenue up and reduces the clients' costs per session. This prompted many to come more often. When our schedules filled and it became necessary to bring a third person to each group, we brought the individual rate to $40 per session, and again the trainer's hourly rose and the client's costs fell. With the addition of each new athlete to the session, the rates fall for the athlete and rise for the trainer, and it all works perfectly unless there's a perceived reduction in attention.

All the demands on the trainer skyrocket in this situation however. Attention, enthusiasm, voice projection, and engagement all have to escalate. It is an acquired skill–an art, really. Our goal is to give so much attention and "in your face" presence to each participant that each is actually grateful that he did not get more attention. The essential shift is that the level of scrutiny and criticism is ratcheted up along with the rate of praise and input for each client. The trainer becomes extremely busy. There is no way a new trainer can walk into this environment and do well. (Imagine the decline in standards for those trainers who are participating in their classes while trying to lead them. We see this too often, and the training is always substandard.)

Within two years we had morphed our one-on-one practice to all group classes without increasing the number of hours we worked each week, although we both kept a couple of choice one-on-one clients. We charged $15 per class and averaged 10 to 15 athletes per session.

This substantially raised our income. It also gave a much-noticed boost to the stability of our practice. Seasonal fluctuations due to summer and Christmas vaca-

The pursuit of excellence is the heart of our business plan."

–COACH GLASSMAN

tions largely disappeared. With a one-on-one practice, when three clients you see two or three times per week are, by coincidence, on vacation simultaneously, income takes a hit. Not so with group classes.

At the same time we started converting our practice from one-on-one to group classes we launched CrossFit.com. The launch of the website was motivated by the same commitment to client and efficacy that motivated our training. We were looking not to increase our revenues but to favorably impact more people with our training. The difference might seem inconsequential, but the public clearly knows the difference.

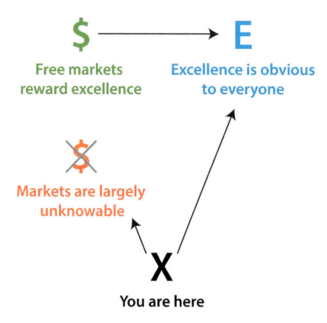

Figure 1. Free Markets Reward Those Who Achieve Excellence.

The group classes, the CrossFit.com website, the CrossFit Journal, our seminars, and our affiliate program were all introduced to bring more quality training to more people. Each of these additions also increased CrossFit's value for everyone involved. It was our original one-on-one clients who initially came to and benefited from the group classes, subscribed to the journal, visited the website, and attended the seminars. Every CrossFit expansion has served the entire community.

We are in pursuit not of money but of excellence. The difference, we believe, is the difference between success and failure. The pursuit of excellence is the heart of our business plan.

Money is, for many, elusive because markets are unknowable. But while markets are unknowable, excellence is obvious to most everyone, especially free, and large, markets.

If you can accept the three premises that:
- Markets are largely unknowable
- Excellence is obvious to everyone, and
- Free markets reward excellence

it becomes obvious that the most effective business plan comes from achieving excellence and letting the market bring the money to you (Figure 1). The efficiency and effectiveness of this paradigm is breathtaking.

We have used the pursuit of excellence to guide our every move. For instance, when we were considering the last expansion of CrossFit Santa Cruz we could not determine whether it would be financially feasible or not. The variables were too numerous and the assumptions too uncertain to convince any accountant of the wisdom of expansion, but when we asked the simple question, "Will it improve the quality of the programming and the training experience?" the answer was a resounding "Yes!" On expansion, the CrossFit Santa Cruz numbers tripled within six months and the extra space allowed for some refinements and additions to our programming that would not have been possible otherwise.

As our seminars, journal, website, and affiliate program grew, we handed off the group classes to a new generation of CrossFit trainers who now cover most of the overhead costs of CrossFit Santa Cruz. This has afforded us time and opportunity to commit more energy and resources to new projects that support and develop the CrossFit community. ∎

CROSSFIT LEVEL 1 TRAINER CERTIFICATE LICENSE AGREEMENT IN PLAIN ENGLISH

Following the successful completion of the CrossFit Level 1 Certificate Course and obtaining a passing score on the CrossFit Level 1 Certificate Course examination, you must agree to the CrossFit Level 1 Trainer Certificate License Agreement ("Agreement"). Be sure to read it thoroughly to gain a clear understanding of what is permitted and prohibited as a CrossFit Level 1 Trainer ("CF-L1"). This document will provide a summary of the Agreement in laymen's terms, although you are responsible for everything required under the full Agreement.

First, it is important to understand the difference between the CrossFit® methodology, and the CrossFit® brand. While the CrossFit® methodology is free to use and to follow on CrossFit.com (and has been for over a decade), the CrossFit® brand name is not free. Even as a CF-L1, you cannot use the CrossFit® brand name to advertise, market, promote, or solicit business or service in any way. If you do, you will be in breach of the Agreement and potentially liable for trademark infringement under Federal Law.

To obtain a license to advertise, market, promote, and solicit business for CrossFit® training (i.e., advertise using the CrossFit® brand name), you must become a licensed CrossFit, Inc. affiliate. Affiliation is described in detail on CrossFit.com, but in summary, you must submit an application (and be accepted) and pay the affiliation fee each year.

As a CF-L1, you may only use the terms "CrossFit Level 1 Trainer" or "CF-L1 Trainer" on a resume, business card, or in a trainer biography on a website. Nothing more is permitted regarding use of the CrossFit® brand name including use of the title "Certified" CrossFit Trainer (which is reserved for CrossFit Level 3 Coaches and above). You can, however, train yourself, teach your friends for free, and introduce the methodology to others, but you cannot use the CrossFit® brand name or CrossFit® copyrighted material (such as this CrossFit Level 1 Training Guide or Participant Handbook) to market your services.

Finally, as a CF-L1, you are required under the Agreement to uphold the highest standards of ethics and behavior; actions that reflect unfavorably on CrossFit, Inc. constitute a breach of the Agreement.

Our legal department aggressively pursues any unlicensed use of the CrossFit® brand name and CrossFit® copyrighted material everywhere in the world. If you are unsure of the appropriate use of the CrossFit® brand name, please contact legalintake@crossfit.com. To report suspected unlicensed use of the CrossFit® brand name, please fill out a form at crossfit.com/iptheft. ▪

FREQUENTLY ASKED QUESTIONS

Can I teach "CrossFit" classes with a CrossFit Level 1 Trainer Certificate?

If you are teaching at a licensed affiliate, you may teach CrossFit® classes and advertise that you are a CF-L1 at that affiliate. If you are not at a licensed affiliate, such as at a commercial gym, you cannot use the CrossFit® brand name in any way to advertise your classes.

If I am a CF-L1, can I advertise or market training similar to CrossFit without using the CrossFit® name?

As a CF-L1, you may use the CrossFit® methodology and you may train people on your own, but only affiliation entitles you to use the CrossFit® trademark (and other CrossFit, Inc. protected intellectual property) to describe your own programming and advertise your services as "CrossFit." To learn more about becoming a licensed affiliate, visit CrossFit.com.

If I am a CF-L1, can I tell my clients we are doing "CrossFit" without advertising it in any written or marketing materials?

No. Word-of-mouth marketing of CrossFit® training is not permitted without first becoming an affiliate. As a CF-L1, you may use the CrossFit® methodology and you may train people on your own, but only affiliation entitles you to use the CrossFit® trademark to describe your own programming, even by word of mouth.

If I hold a CrossFit Level 1 Trainer Certificate but do not work at an affiliate, how can I promote that I do CrossFit® training without opening a gym?

A personal trainer with a CrossFit Level 1 Trainer Certificate who trains clients in non-affiliate locations (e.g., at their homes, commercial gyms) cannot use the CrossFit® trademark without becoming an affiliate. See above. However, as outlined in the Agreement, a CF-L1 may state their credential on a business card, resume, or trainer biography.

Can I call myself a "Certified" CrossFit Trainer?

No. This terminology is reserved for CrossFit Level 3 trainers and above. The correct terminology to describe your certificate is "CrossFit Level 1 Trainer" or "CF-L1 Trainer."

What does obtaining a CrossFit Level 1 Trainer Certificate afford an individual beyond a designation?

Your status as a CF-L1 means you will be listed in the CrossFit Trainer Directory, an online database for the public to locate licensed CrossFit® trainers.

What does obtaining a CrossFit Level 1 Trainer Certificate afford an individual for furthering his or her education?

The CrossFit Level 1 Trainer Certificate is a prerequisite for more advanced courses offered by CrossFit, Inc., including the CrossFit® Level 2 Certificate Course.

What else am I required to do under the Agreement?

We require all CF-L1s to uphold the highest standards of ethics and behavior; actions that reflect unfavorably on CrossFit, Inc. constitute a breach of the Agreement.

How do I contact CrossFit, Inc. if I suspect other CF-L1s are misusing the CrossFit® brand name?

Please fill out the reporting form at crossfit.com/iptheft. Our legal department aggressively pursues any unlicensed use of the CrossFit® brand name and CrossFit® copyrighted material everywhere in the world. ▪

CROSSFIT CREDENTIALS

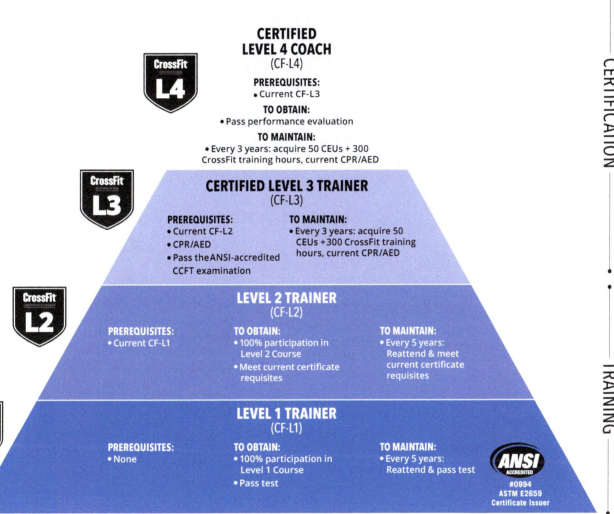

**CERTIFIED
LEVEL 4 COACH**
(CF-L4)

PREREQUISITES:
• Current CF-L3

TO OBTAIN:
• Pass performance evaluation

TO MAINTAIN:
• Every 3 years: acquire 50 CEUs + 300
CrossFit training hours, current CPR/AED

CERTIFIED LEVEL 3 TRAINER
(CF-L3)

PREREQUISITES:
• Current CF-L2
• CPR/AED
• Pass the ANSI-accredited
  CCFT examination

TO MAINTAIN:
• Every 3 years: acquire 50
  CEUs +300 CrossFit training
  hours, current CPR/AED

LEVEL 2 TRAINER
(CF-L2)

PREREQUISITES:
• Current CF-L1

TO OBTAIN:
• 100% participation in
  Level 2 Course
• Meet current certificate
  requisites

TO MAINTAIN:
• Every 5 years:
  Reattend & meet
  current certificate
  requisites

LEVEL 1 TRAINER
(CF-L1)

PREREQUISITES:
• None

TO OBTAIN:
• 100% participation in
  Level 1 Course
• Pass test

TO MAINTAIN:
• Every 5 years:
  Reattend & pass test

ANSI
ACCREDITED
#0994
ASTM E2659
Certificate Issuer

CERTIFICATION

TRAINING

Visit CrossFit.com to learn more about CrossFit's credentials.

NINE FOUNDATIONAL MOVEMENTS SUMMARY

Effective coaching can be measured as a trainer's capacity in six areas: teaching, seeing, correcting, group management, presence and attitude, and demonstration. This section helps participants learn the fundamentals of the first three: teaching, seeing, and correcting the nine foundational movements of the Level 1 Certificate Course.

The nine foundational movements of the Level 1 Course are:
- The Air Squat
- The Front Squat
- The Overhead Squat
- The Shoulder Press
- The Push Press
- The Push Jerk
- The Deadlift
- The Sumo Deadlift High Pull
- The Medicine-Ball Clean

Teaching requires knowing the necessary points of performance for proper execution, including set-up and finish positions. Seeing builds on this knowledge by requiring the trainer to assess these points of performance (and deviation from them) in real time. Correcting is the ability to improve a client's mechanics to better adhere to the points of performance.

Each movement has at least two sections: 1) Points of Performance; and 2) Common Faults and Corrections. Where applicable, some movements also have a third section: 3) Teaching Progression. These progressions break complex movements down into simple steps that focus on developing the primary points of performance in the full movement.

This section is not meant to serve as an exhaustive resource of all the knowledge, teaching progressions, or possible corrections when coaching movements. Rather, it is a sufficient introductory guide to support the development of new trainers. ∎

THE AIR SQUAT

The air squat is the cornerstone movement of CrossFit and is foundational to the front squat and overhead squat. The air squat raises one's center of mass from a seated to standing position.

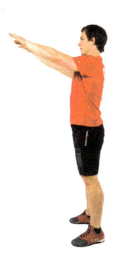
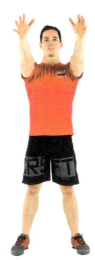

1. SET-UP

- Shoulder-width stance.

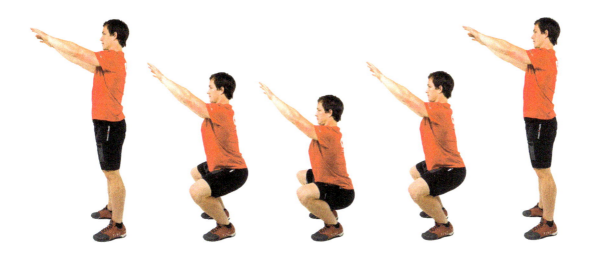

2. EXECUTION

- Hips descend back and down.
- Lumbar curve maintained.
- Knees in line with toes.
- Hips descend lower than knees.
- Heels down.

3. FINISH

- Complete at full hip and knee extension.

THE AIR SQUAT COMMON FAULTS AND CORRECTIONS

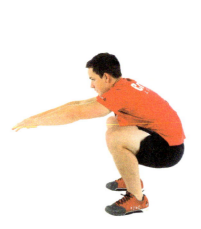

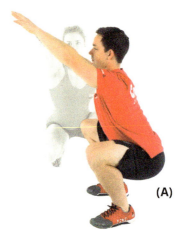

FAULT:

- Loss of a neutral position due to flexion in lumbar spine.

CORRECTIONS:

- Cue the athlete to lift the chest.
- Have the athlete raise the arms as he or she descends to the bottom of the squat. **(A)**

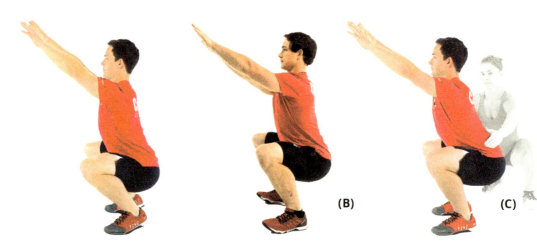

FAULT:

- Weight on toes or shifting to toes.

CORRECTIONS:

- Have the athlete exaggerate weight on the heels by lifting the toes slightly throughout the entire movement. **(B)**
- Give a tactile cue to push the hips back and down. **(C)**

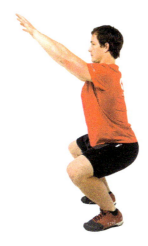

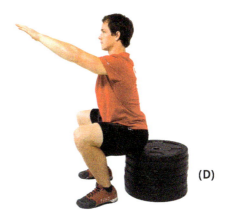

(D)

FAULT:

- Not going low enough.

CORRECTIONS:

- Cue "Lower!" and do not relent.
- Have the athlete squat to a target that places the hip crease lower than the knee to develop awareness of depth. **(D)**

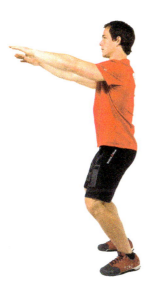

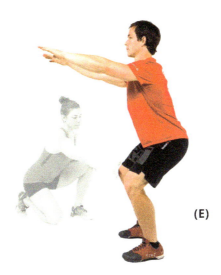

(E)

FAULT:

- Improper line of action: hips do not travel back, knees move excessively forward placing weight on the toes.

CORRECTIONS:

- Give a tactile cue to push the hips back and down.
- Block the knees' forward travel with the hand at the initiation of the descent to encourage movement of the hips. **(E)**

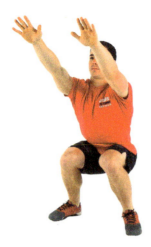
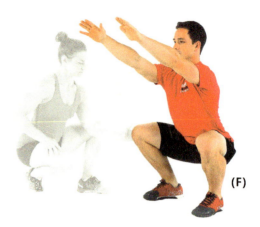

(F)

FAULT:

- Knees not tracking in line with toes, which usually causes them to roll inside the feet.

CORRECTIONS:

- Cue "Push your knees out" or "Spread the ground apart with your feet."
- Use a target on the outside of the knee for the athlete to reach. **(F)**

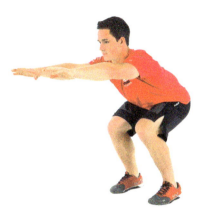 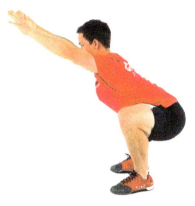

FAULT:

- Multiple-fault squat: Inability to
  - Maintain lumbar curve;
  - Keep weight on the heels;
  - Keep the knees tracking in line with the feet; and
  - Get to depth all at the same time.

FAULT:

- Immature squat: All points of performance are maintained but the athlete has to cantilever forward excessively onto the quads to maintain balance.

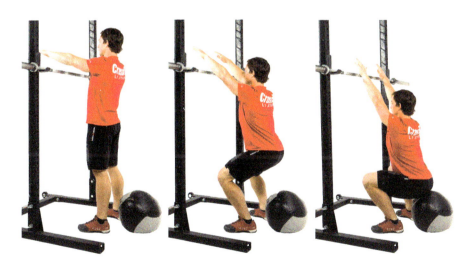

CORRECTION:

- Squat Therapy: Set the athlete facing a wall or racked bar with a target at depth. Set him or her in the proper stance, with heels to the box, chest close to wall. Have the athlete squat to the box slowly, maintaining control and weight on the heels.

THE FRONT SQUAT

The points of performance, common faults, and corrections carry over from the air squat. The new element of the front squat is the addition of a loaded barbell to the front of the body. The barbell is supported by the torso in the front-rack position.

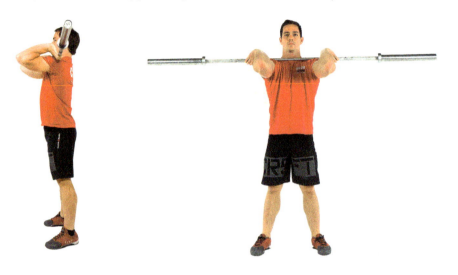

1. SET-UP

- Shoulder-width stance.
- Loose fingertip grip on the bar.
- Hands just outside shoulders.
- Elbows high (upper arm parallel to the ground).

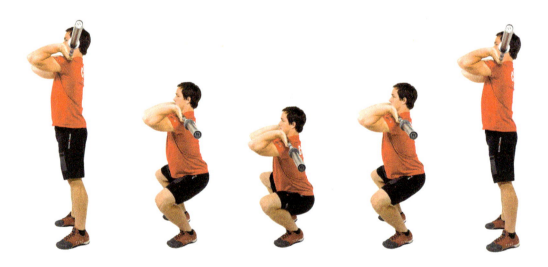

2. EXECUTION

- Hips descend back and down.
- Lumbar curve maintained.
- Knees in line with toes.
- Hips descend lower than knees.
- Heels down.

3. FINISH

- Complete at full hip and knee extension.

THE FRONT SQUAT COMMON FAULTS AND CORRECTIONS

All faults and corrections from the air squat apply to this movement, plus the following:

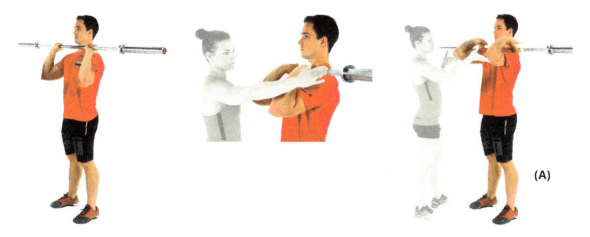

(A)

FAULT:

- Improper rack position where the bar is not in contact with the torso.

CORRECTIONS:

- Ensure the athlete has an open grip and the bar is resting on the fingertips.
- Cue "Elbows high!"
- Manually adjust the rack position. **(A)**

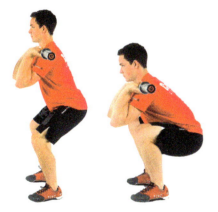
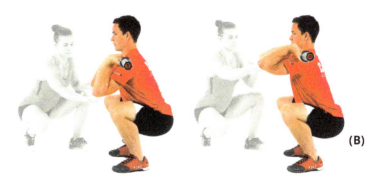

(B)

FAULT:

- Elbows drop during the squat.

CORRECTIONS:

- Encourage the athlete to move their elbows away from the trainer's hands. **(B)**
- Cue "Elbows up!" and encourage athlete to lift the chest.

THE OVERHEAD SQUAT

The points of performance, common faults, and corrections carry over from the air squat. The new element in the overhead squat is a load added in the overhead position.

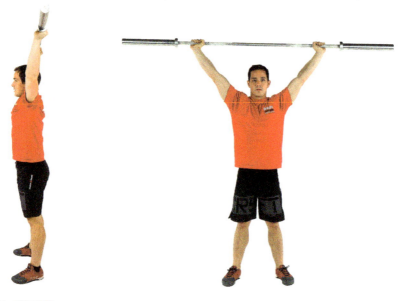

1. SET-UP

- Shoulder-width stance.
- Shoulders push up into the bar.
- Arms extended.

- Wide grip on the bar (wide enough to perform a pass-through).
- Armpits face forward.

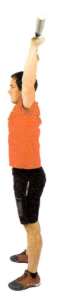
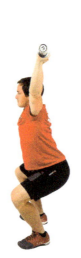
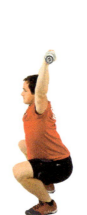
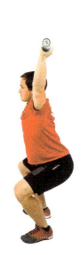
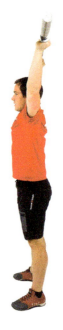

2. EXECUTION

- Hips descend back and down.
- Knees in line with toes.
- Lumbar curve maintained.

- Hips descend lower than knees.
- Heels down.
- Bar moves over the middle of the foot.

3. FINISH

- Complete at full hip and knee extension.

THE OVERHEAD SQUAT COMMON FAULTS AND CORRECTIONS

All faults and corrections from the air squat apply to this movement, plus the following:

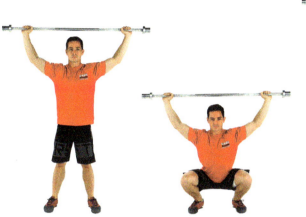

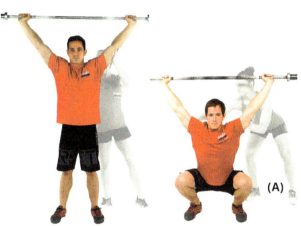

FAULT:

- Inactive overhead position due to flexed elbows and/or inactive shoulders.

CORRECTIONS:

- Cue athlete to press the bar up.
- Use a tactile cue to push the elbows straight, shoulders up, and armpits forward. **(A)**

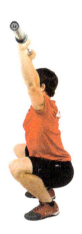

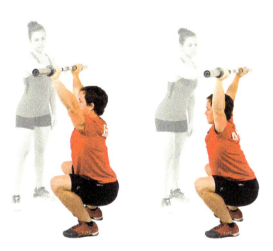

FAULT:

- Bar moves forward of the frontal plane.

CORRECTION:

- Cue the athlete to press the bar up and pull it back over midfoot or slightly behind the frontal plane.

THE SHOULDER PRESS

The shoulder press is foundational to all the overhead lifts. The key elements of this lift are a neutral spine, straight bar path and correct overhead position.

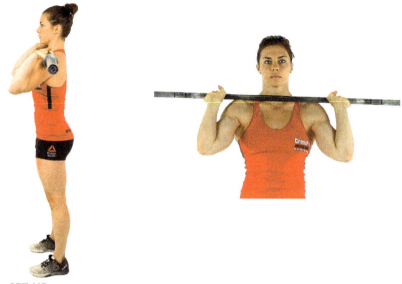

1. SET-UP

- Hip-width stance.
- Elbows slightly in front of the bar.
- Hands just outside shoulders.
- Full grip on the bar.
- Bar rests on torso.

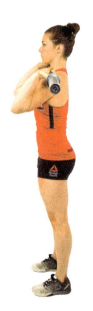
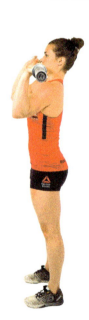
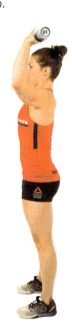
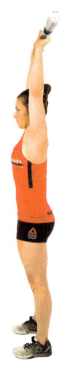

2. EXECUTION

- Spine neutral and legs extended.
- Heels down.
- Bar moves over the middle of the foot.
- Shoulders push up into the bar.

3. FINISH

- Complete at full arm extension.

THE SHOULDER PRESS COMMON FAULTS AND CORRECTIONS

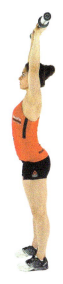

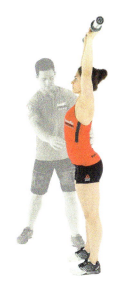

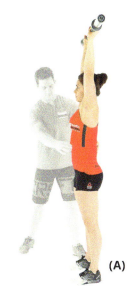

(A)

FAULT:

- Overextending the spine with the ribs sticking out.

CORRECTIONS:

- Have the athlete tighten the abdominals by pulling the rib cage down (be sure to check the overhead position again after this fix). **(A)**
- Have the athlete use a slightly wider grip if needed, until flexibility improves.

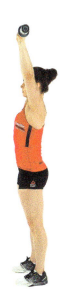

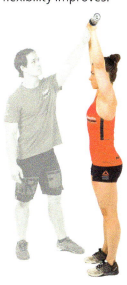

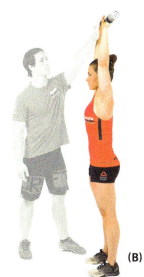

(B)

FAULT:

- Bar finishes forward of frontal plane.

CORRECTIONS:

- Cue the athlete to press up and pull back on the bar as it travels overhead.
- Use a tactile cue and gently push the bar back into the correct position. **(B)**

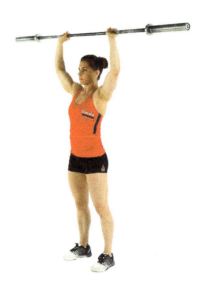

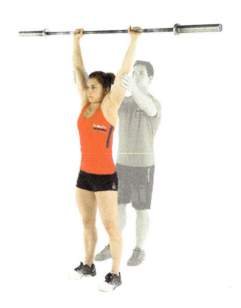

FAULT:

- Elbows are bent or shoulders are not active.

CORRECTION:

- Cue "Press up!" and use a tactile cue to lock out the elbows and push the shoulders up.

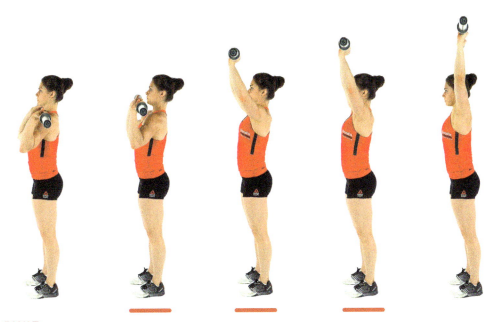

FAULT:

- Bar arcs out around the face instead of moving straight up and following the frontal plane.

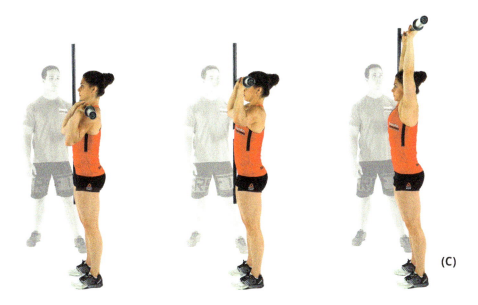

(C)

CORRECTIONS:

- Cue the athlete to pull the head back and out of the way of the bar.
- Check that elbows are not too low in the set-up.
- Block the forward travel of the bar with another object, such as a piece of PVC. **(C)**

183 |

THE PUSH PRESS

The push press builds on the shoulder press. The set-up, bar path and spinal and overhead positions are the same as in the shoulder press. Unique to the push press is a vertical dip of the torso followed by a rapid extension of the hips, which adds velocity to the movement.

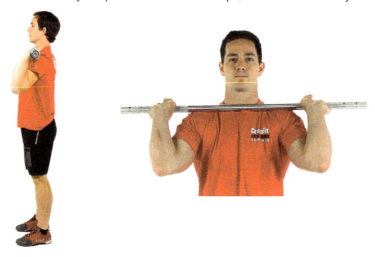

1. SET-UP

- Hip-width stance.
- Elbows slightly in front of the bar.
- Hands just outside shoulders.
- Full grip on the bar.
- Bar rests on torso.

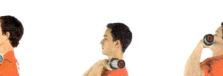
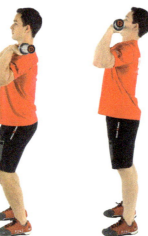
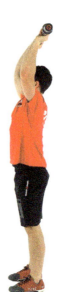
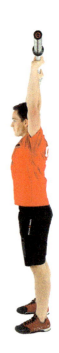

2. EXECUTION

- Torso remains vertical as hips and knees flex in the dip.
- Hips and legs extend, then arms press.
- Heels remain down until hips and knees extend.
- Bar moves over the middle of the foot.

3. FINISH

- Complete at full hip, knee, and arm extension.

THE PUSH PRESS TEACHING PROGRESSION

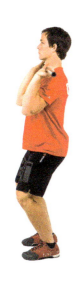
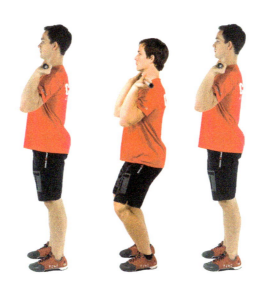

STEP 1:
- Dip and hold.

STEP 2:
- Dip-drive, slow.

STEP 3:
- Dip-drive, fast.

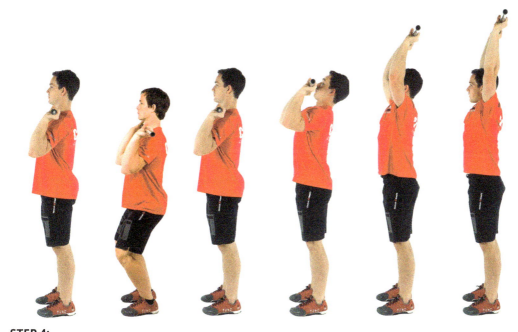

STEP 4:
- Full push press.

THE PUSH PRESS COMMON FAULTS AND CORRECTIONS

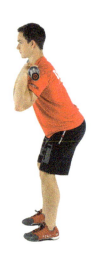 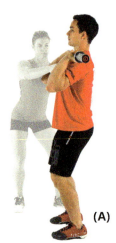

(A)   (B)

FAULT:

- Forward inclination of the chest during the dip.

CORRECTIONS:

- Have the athlete hold the dip. Manually adjust him or her to an upright position. **(A)**
- Cue a shorter dip.
- Cue "Knees forward."
- Stand in front of athlete to prevent the chest from coming forward.
- Dip Therapy: Have the athlete stand against a target with hips and shoulder blades touching the target (heels slightly away). Then have the athlete dip and drive while keeping the hips and shoulders in contact with the target. **(B)**

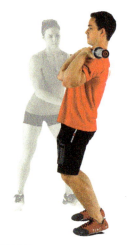 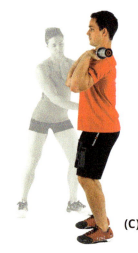

(C)

FAULT:

- Muted hips: hips push forward during the dip.

CORRECTIONS:

- Use a tactile cue to help the athlete create flexion of the hip in the dip. **(C)**
- Cue "Push the hips back slightly."

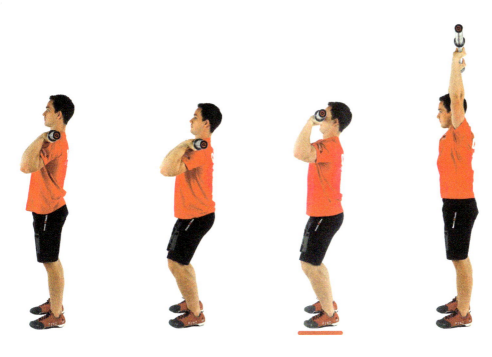

FAULT:
- Pressing early: press begins before the hip extends.

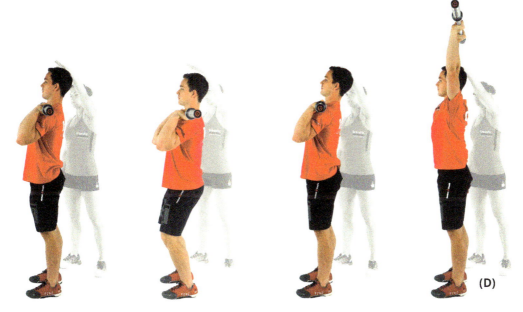

(D)

CORRECTIONS:
- Take the athlete back in the teaching progression to perform two dip-drives before adding the press.
- Place your hand at the top of the athlete's head when fully standing; keep it at that height and then ask the athlete to hit your hand during the drive before pressing. **(D)**

THE PUSH JERK

The push jerk builds on both the shoulder press and push press. The set-up, bar path and spinal and overhead positions are the same, as are the dip and drive. Unique to the push jerk is the press under the bar. After extension of the hip, the athlete presses against the bar and receives the lift in a partial overhead squat before standing to finish the lift.

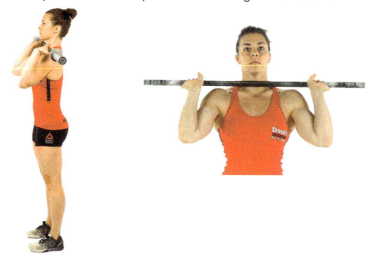

1. SET-UP

- Hip-width stance.
- Elbows slightly in front of the bar.

- Hands just outside shoulders.
- Full grip on the bar.
- Bar rests on torso.

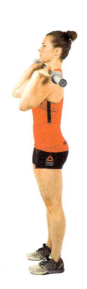
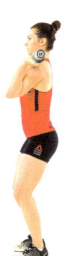
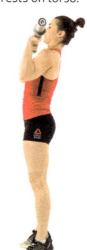
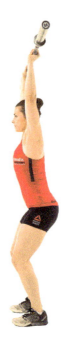
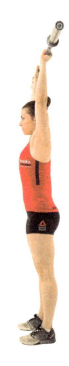

2. EXECUTION

- Bar rests on torso.
- Torso remains vertical as hips and knees flex in the dip.

- Heels stay down until hips and knees extend.
- Hips and knees extend rapidly, then arms press to drive under the bar.

3. FINISH

- Complete at full hip, knee, and arm extension.

THE PUSH JERK TEACHING PROGRESSION

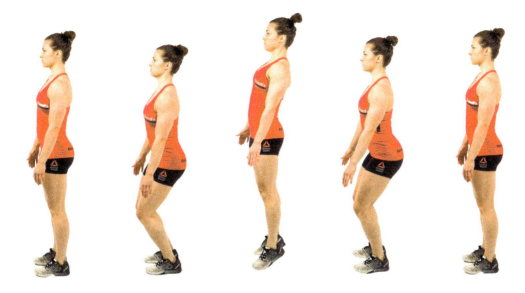

STEP 1:

- Jump and land with hands at sides. Stick the landing before standing.

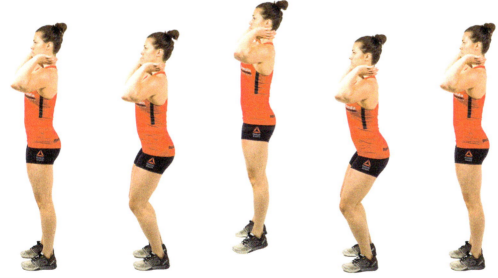

STEP 2:

- Jump and land with hands at shoulders. Stick the landing before standing.

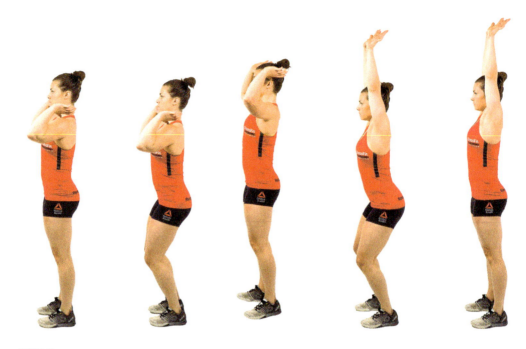

STEP 3:

- Jump and extend the arms after the hip opens. Stick the landing before standing with arms overhead.

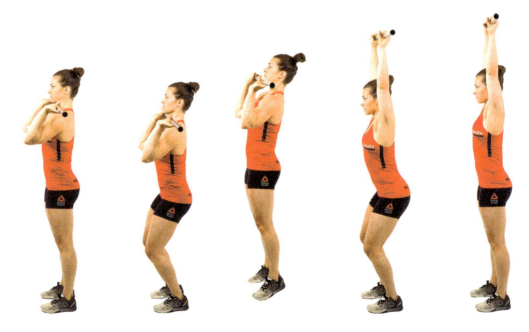

STEP 4:

- With the PVC in hands, complete the full push jerk.

THE PUSH JERK COMMON FAULTS AND CORRECTIONS

All faults and corrections from the shoulder press and push press apply to this movement, plus the following:

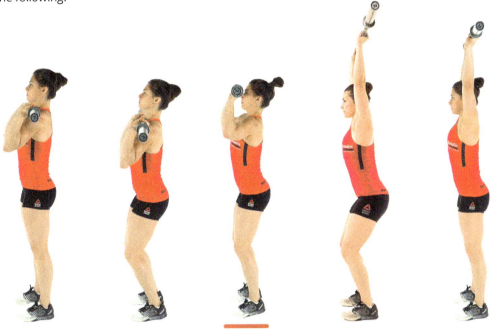

FAULT:

- Lack of full hip extension.

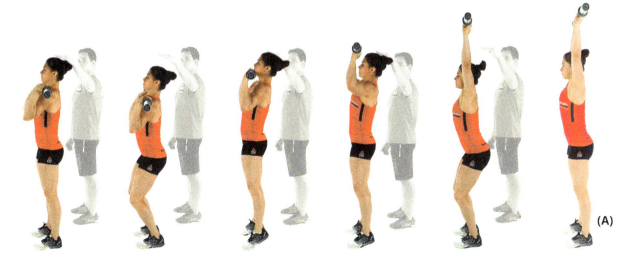

(A)

CORRECTIONS:

- Cue "Jump higher."
- Place your hand at the top of the athlete's head when fully standing; keep it at that height and then ask the athlete to hit your hand during the drive. **(A)**
- Take the athlete back to steps 1-3 of the teaching progression. Have the athlete focus on reaching hip extension before moving on to the next step.
- Encourage the athlete to squeeze the glutes and quads before pressing under.

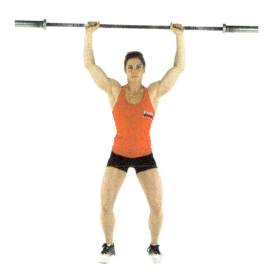

FAULT:

- Poor/inactive overhead position (particularly when receiving the bar).

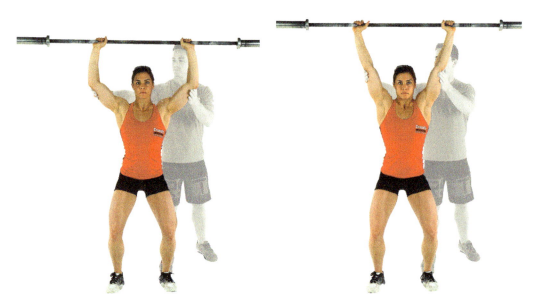

CORRECTION:

- Cue the athlete to press up on the bar while in the receiving position, before standing to extension.

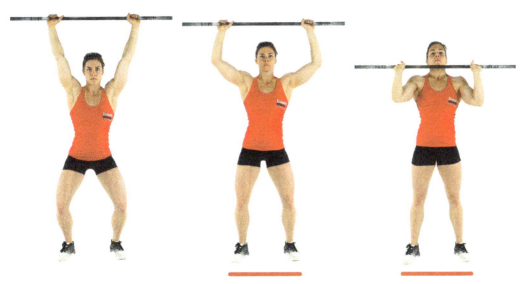

FAULT:

- Lowering the bar before standing all the way up.

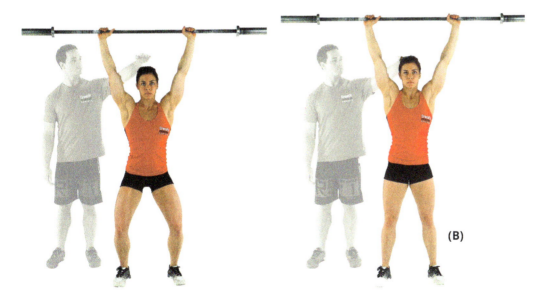

(B)

CORRECTIONS:

- Cue the athlete to keep the bar overhead until hips and knees are fully extended.
- Use a tactile cue: hold your hand over the athlete's head and instruct him or her to hit the hand before lowering the bar. **(B)**

THE DEADLIFT

The deadlift is foundational to all pulling lifts. For proper execution of the deadlift, the spine should be neutral at all times and the object should be kept close to the frontal plane throughout the range of motion.

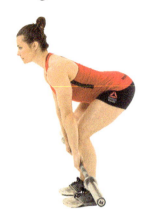 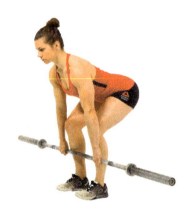

1. SET-UP

- Hip-to-shoulder-width stance.
- Hands just outside hips.
- Eyes on the horizon.

- Full grip on the bar.
- Shoulders slightly in front of or over the bar.
- Arms straight and bar in contact with the shins.

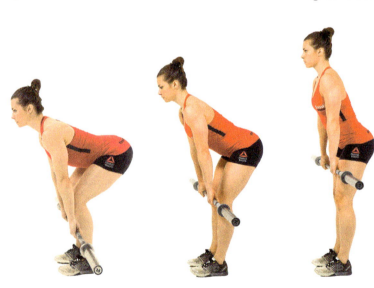 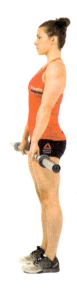

2. EXECUTION

- Lumbar curve maintained.
- Hips and shoulders rise at the same rate until the bar passes the knee.
- Hips then open.
- Bar moves over the middle of the foot.
- Heels down.

3. FINISH

- Complete at full hip and knee extension.

THE DEADLIFT COMMON FAULTS AND CORRECTIONS

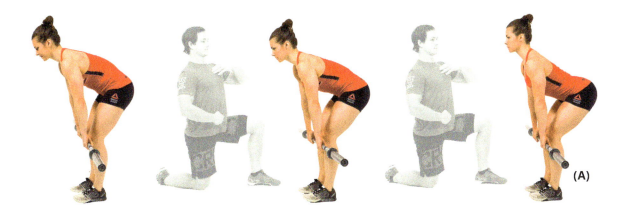

FAULT:

- Loss of lumbar curve due to flexion of the spine.

CORRECTIONS:

- Abort current lift and decrease the load to where the lumbar curve can be maintained.
- At a lower weight, cue the athlete to "lift the chest" and do not relent. **(A)**

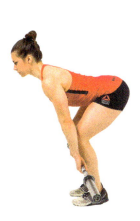
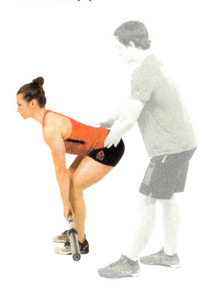

FAULT:

- Weight on, or shifting, to toes.

CORRECTION:

- Have the athlete pull the hips back and settle on the heels. Have him or her focus on driving through heels.

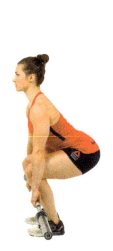
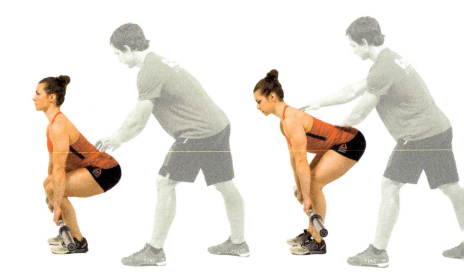

FAULT:

- Shoulders behind bar in set-up.

CORRECTION:

- Raise the hips to move the shoulders over, or slightly in front of, the bar.

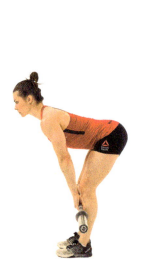
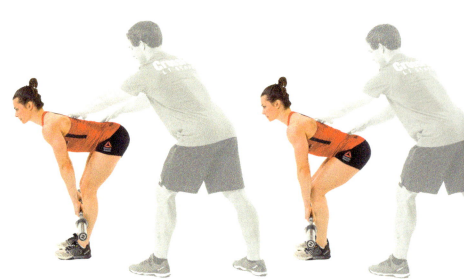

FAULT:

- Hips too high in set-up.

CORRECTION:

- Lower the hips to move the shoulders over, or slightly in front of, the bar.

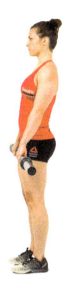 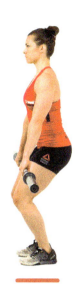 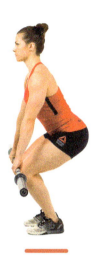

FAULT:

- Hips do not move back to initiate the descent.

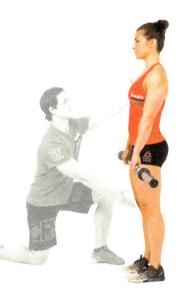 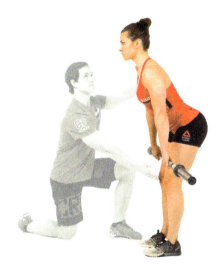 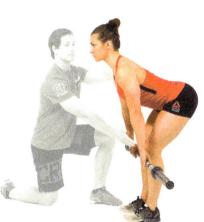

CORRECTION:

- Cue the athlete to initiate the return by pushing the hips back and delaying the knee bend until the bar passes below the knees.

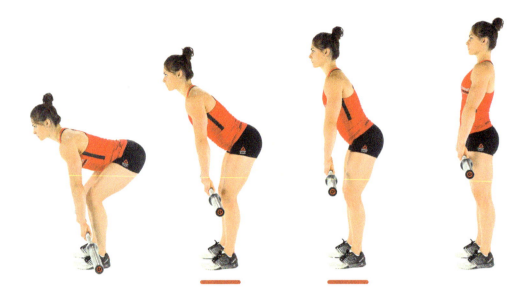

FAULT:

- Bar loses contact with legs.

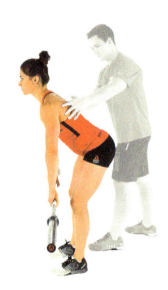

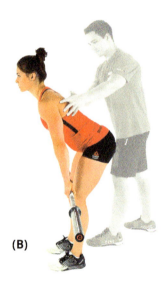

(B)

CORRECTIONS:

- Cue "Pull the bar in to your legs the whole time."
- Use a tactile cue to help engage the upper back. **(B)**

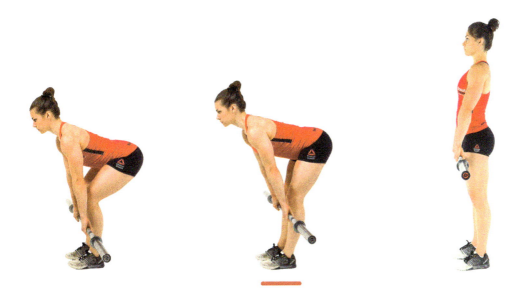

FAULT:
- Hips rise before the chest (stiff-legged deadlift).

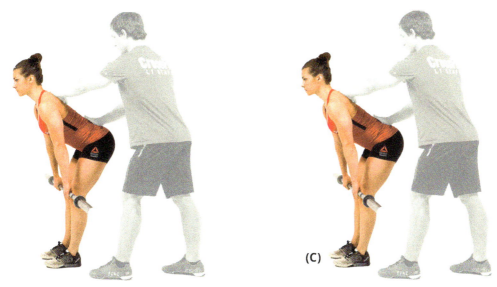

(C)

CORRECTIONS:
- Cue "Lift your chest more aggressively."
- Give a tactile cue at the hips and shoulders so they rise in unison. **(C)**

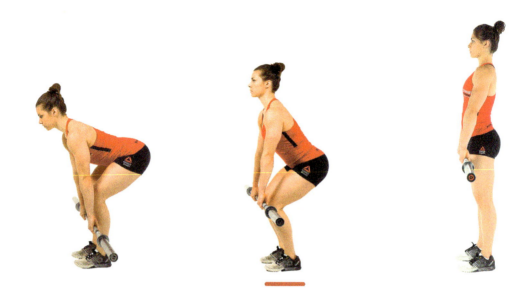

FAULT:

- Shoulders rise without the hips. Bar travels around the knees instead of straight up.

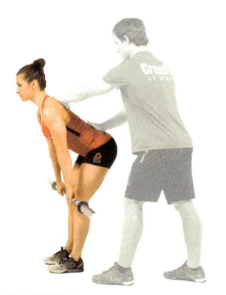
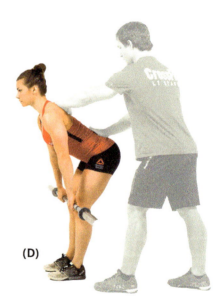

(D)

CORRECTIONS:

- Cue "Push the knees back as your chest rises."
- Be sure the athlete is set up correctly and that the hips are not too low.
- Give a tactile cue at the hips and shoulders so they rise in unison. **(D)**

THE SUMO DEADLIFT HIGH PULL

The sumo deadlift high pull builds on the deadlift but uses a wider stance and a narrower grip. The sumo deadlift high pull also adds velocity and range of motion. This movement is a good example of a core-to-extremity movement: the bar is accelerated by the hips and legs before the arms are engaged to finish the pull.

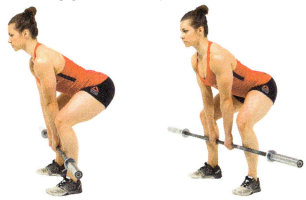

1. SET-UP

- Slightly wider than shoulder-width stance.
- Hands inside legs with a full grip on the bar.
- Shoulders slightly in front of or over the bar.
- Knees in line with toes.
- Arms straight and bar in contact with the shins.
- Eyes on the horizon.

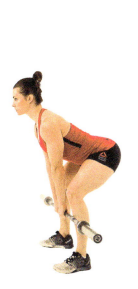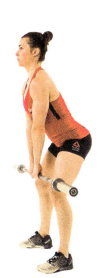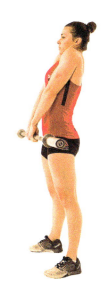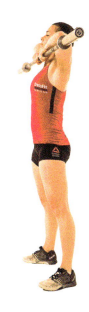

2. EXECUTION

- Lumbar curve maintained.
- Hips and shoulders rise at the same rate until the bar passes the knee.
- Hips then extend rapidly.
- Heels down until hips and legs extend.
- Shoulders shrug, then the arms pull.
- Elbows move high and outside.
- Bar moves over the middle of the foot.

3. FINISH

- Complete at full hip and knee extension with the bar pulled under the chin.

THE SUMO DEADLIFT HIGH PULL TEACHING PROGRESSION

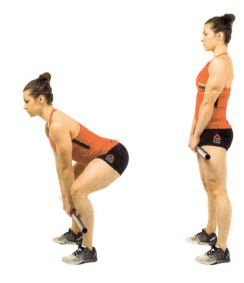

STEP 1:

- Sumo deadlift.

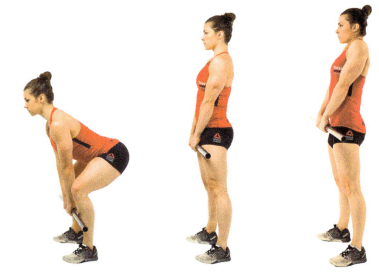

STEP 2:

- Sumo deadlift-shrug, slow.

STEP 3:

- Sumo deadlift-shrug, fast.

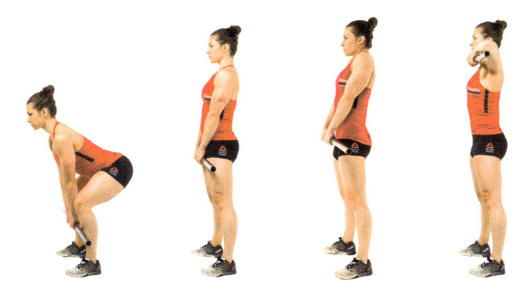

STEP 4:

■ Full sumo deadlift high pull.

THE SUMO DEADLIFT HIGH PULL COMMON FAULTS AND CORRECTIONS

All faults and corrections from the deadlift apply to this movement, plus the following:

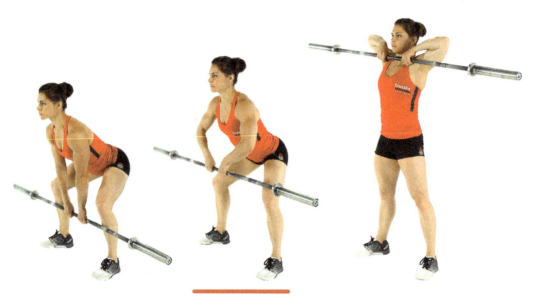

FAULT:

- Pulling early: the shoulders shrug or the arms bend before the hips are completely extended.

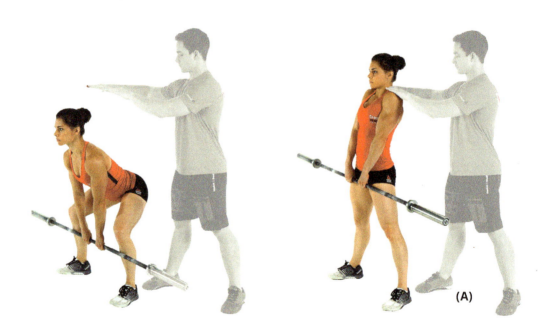

(A)

CORRECTIONS:

- Take the athlete back in the teaching progression to work the deadlift-shrug at a speed that allows correct timing. Once the deadlift-shrug is correct at speed, try two deadlift-shrugs for every one full sumo deadlift high pull.
- Give a tactile cue to have the athlete hit your hands with his or her shoulders before pulling with the arms. **(A)**

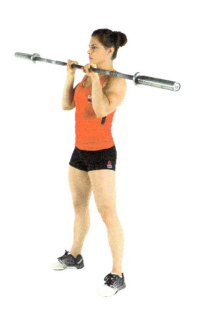

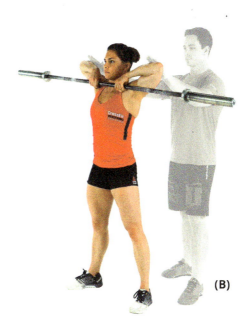

FAULT:

- Athlete pulls with the elbows low and inside.

CORRECTIONS:

- Cue "Elbows high!"
- Give a tactile cue to have the athlete hit your hands where his or her elbows should finish. **(B)**

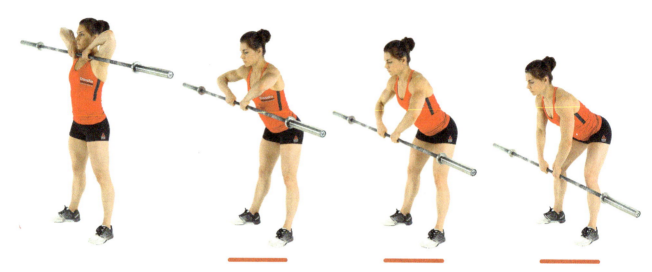

FAULT:

- Incorrect descent (hips flex before the arms extend).

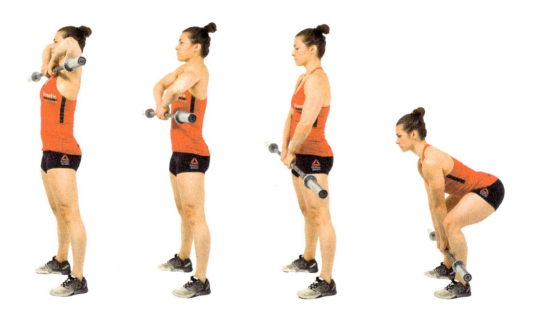

CORRECTION:

- Slow down the movement and have the athlete practice the return in a segmented fashion by extending the arms first before re-introducing speed.

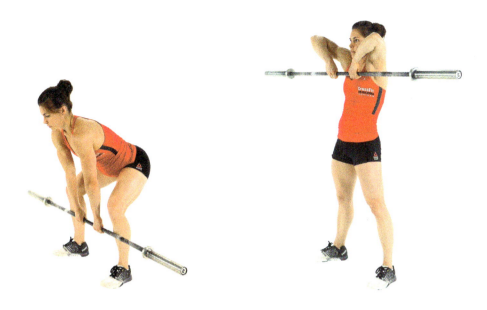

FAULT:

- Shoulders rolling forward in the set-up or during the pull.

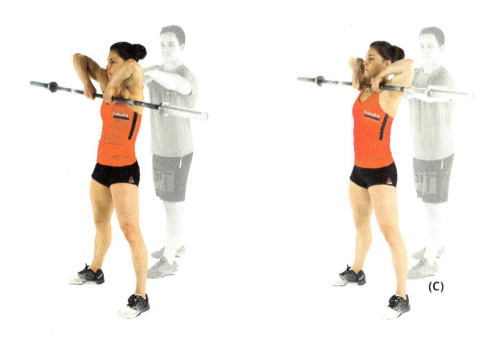

(C)

CORRECTIONS:

- Correct the position in the set-up or at the top of the pull. **(C)**
- Widen the grip and/or reduce the range of motion so the shoulders remain in the proper position.

THE MEDICINE-BALL CLEAN

The medicine-ball clean builds on the deadlift and the sumo deadlift high pull. Unique to the medicine-ball clean is the pull-under, which allows the athlete to bring the object to a position of support (the front-rack position).

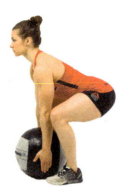 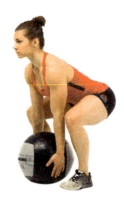

1. SET-UP

- Shoulder-width stance.
- Ball between the feet with palms on the ball.

- Knees in line with toes.
- Shoulders over the ball.
- Eyes on the horizon.

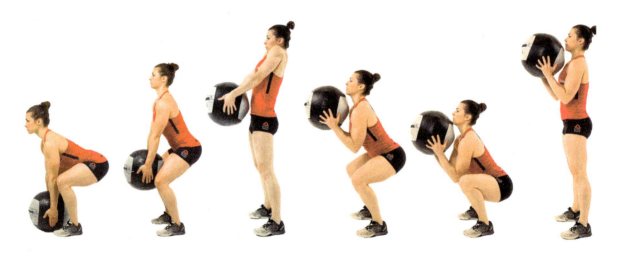

2. EXECUTION

- Lumbar curve maintained.
- Hips extend rapidly.
- Shoulders then shrug.

- Heels down until the hips and knees extend.
- Arms then pull under to the bottom of the squat.
- Ball stays close to the body.

3. FINISH

- Complete at full hip and knee extension with the ball at the rack position.

THE MEDICINE-BALL CLEAN TEACHING PROGRESSION

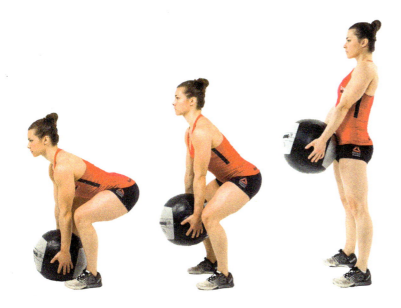

STEP 1:

- Deadlift.

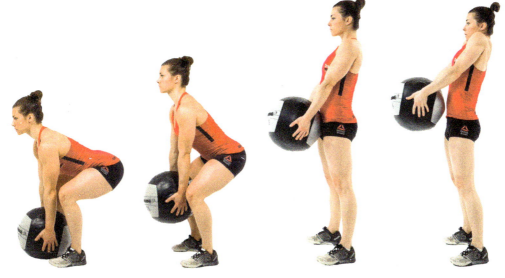

STEP 2:

- Deadlift-shrug, fast.

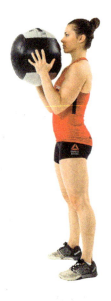
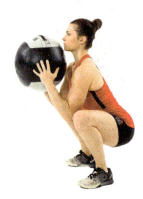

STEP 3:

- Front squat.

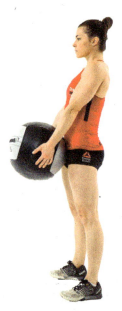
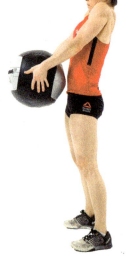
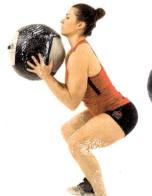
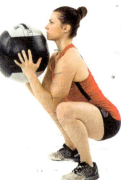

STEP 4:

- Pull-under.

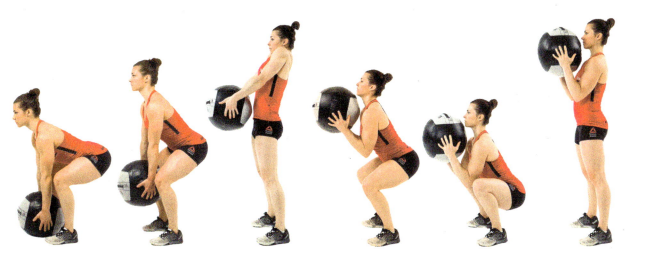

STEP 5:

- Full medicine-ball clean.

THE MEDICINE-BALL CLEAN COMMON FAULTS AND CORRECTIONS

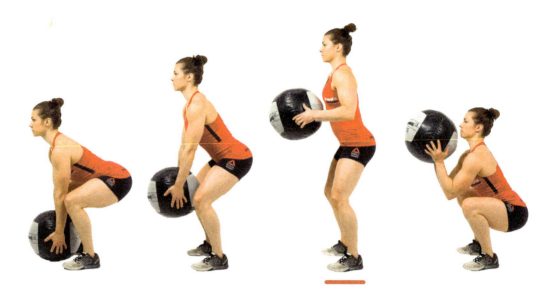

FAULT:

- Lack of full hip extension.

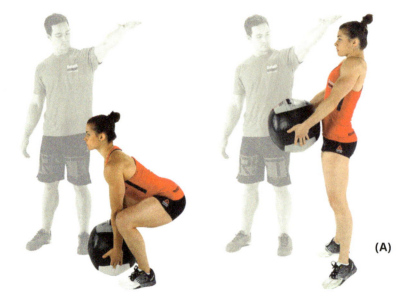

(A)

CORRECTIONS:

- Take athlete back to the teaching progression and have him or her do two deadlift-shrugs for every one medicine-ball clean.
- Give a tactile cue to have the athlete hit your hand with his or her head before pulling under the ball. **(A)**

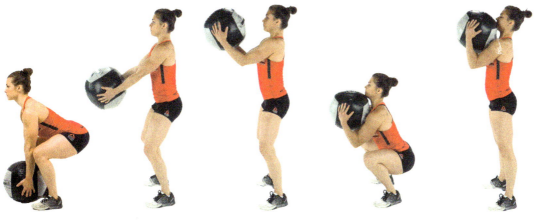

FAULT:

- Curling the ball.

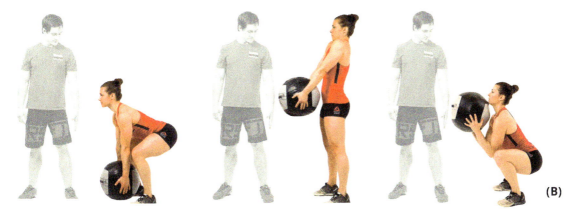

(B)

CORRECTIONS:

- Stand in front of the athlete to block him or her from curling (can also use a wall). **(B)**
- Cue "Elbows high and outside!"

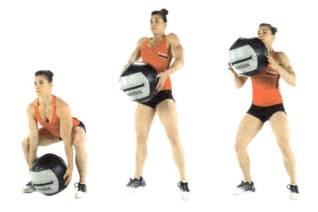

CORRECTION:

- Require the athlete to keep the laces (or any markings) of the ball facing out for the entire movement.

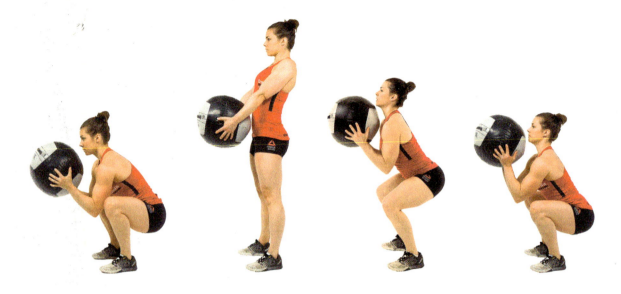

FAULT:

- Collapsing in the receiving position.

CORRECTION:

- Take the athlete back to the teaching progression and have him or her practice the pull-under with sound front squat mechanics.

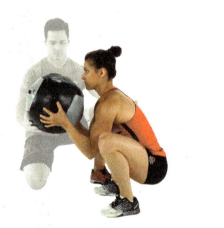
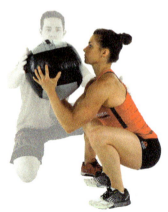

CORRECTION:

- Cue the athlete to lift the chest in the front squat.

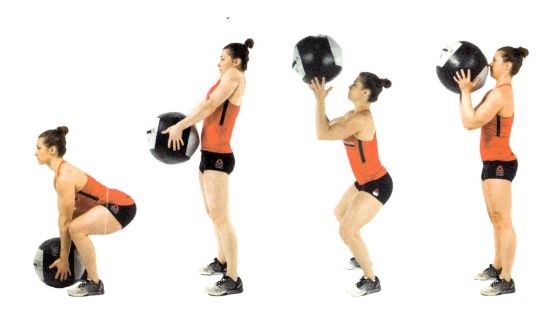

FAULT:

- Receiving too high.

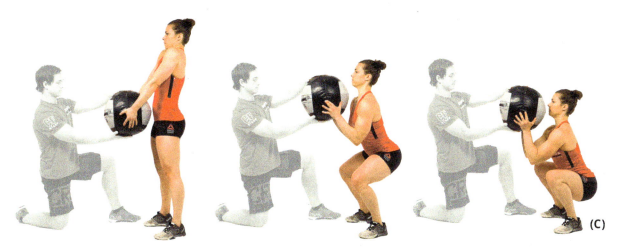

(C)

CORRECTIONS:

- Hold the ball at the peak of the shrug and let the athlete practice the pull-under without moving the ball higher. **(C)**
- Take athlete back to the teaching progression and have him or her practice the pull-under. Have him or her do two pull-unders for every one medicine-ball clean.

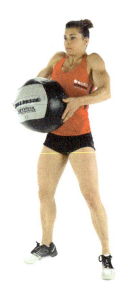 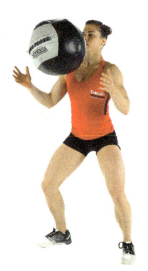 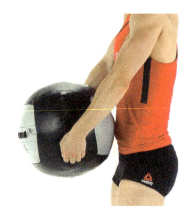

FAULT:

- Tossing or flicking the medicine ball up without pulling under.

CORRECTION:

- Have the athlete hold the ball without the fingers, using palms or fists only.

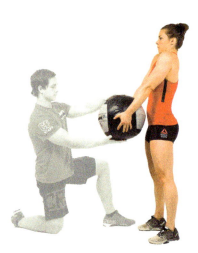 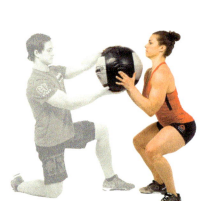 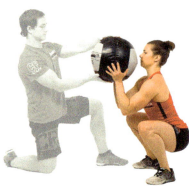

CORRECTION:

- Hold ball at the peak of the shrug and let athlete practice the pull-under to feel the rotation of the hands.

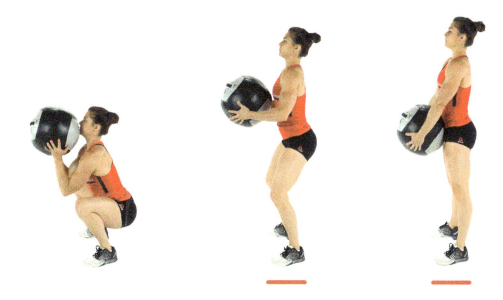

FAULT:

- Not standing up before lowering the weight.

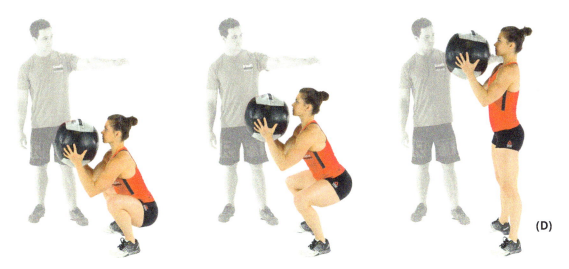

(D)

CORRECTIONS:

- Give a tactile cue to have the athlete keep the ball at the chest until his or her shoulder contacts a target. **(D)**
- Cue the athlete to stand all the way up before lowering the ball from the chest.

FOUR ADDITIONAL MOVEMENTS SUMMARY

The four additional movements of the Level 1 Course are:
- The Pull-up
- The Thruster
- The Muscle-up
- The Snatch

As in the instructions for the nine foundational movements, each movement has three sections: 1) Points of Performance; 2) Common Faults and Corrections; and 3) Teaching Progression.

We teach these movements at the Level 1 Course to improve participants' mechanics and also to provide a teaching method for more complicated movements. ▪

> The most important criterion for exercise selection is neuroendocrine effect. Regardless of your sport or your fitness goals, these moves are the shortest path to success."
>
> –COACH GLASSMAN

THE PULL-UP

The kipping pull-up is CrossFit's default pull-up. It allows the athlete to accomplish more work in less time (higher power) due to the hips assisting the upper-body pull. CrossFit recommends athletes have at least one strict pull-up before performing kipping pull-ups.

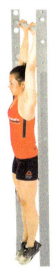 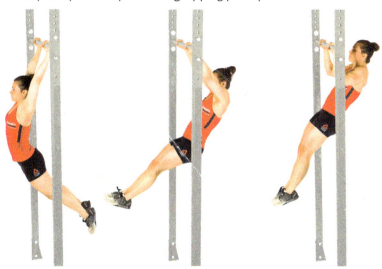

1. SET-UP

- Hands just outside shoulder width.
- Hang with arms extended.

2. EXECUTION

- Initiate kip swing with the shoulders.
- As feet swing forward, push bar straight down with the arms.
- Chest stays up with the eyes forward.

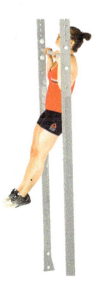 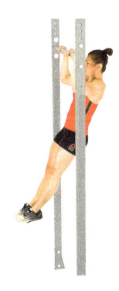 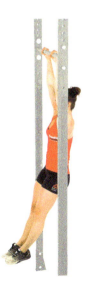 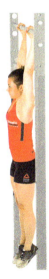

EXECUTION, CONTINUED

- Pull until chin is higher than the bar.
- Push away from the bar to begin the descent.
- Return to full extension to begin the next repetition.

THE PULL-UP TEACHING PROGRESSION

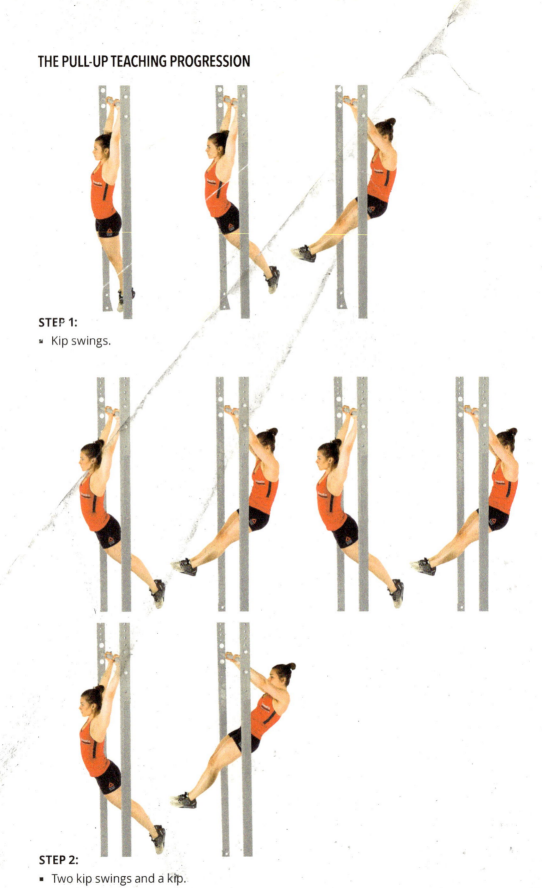

STEP 1:
- Kip swings.

STEP 2:
- Two kip swings and a kip.

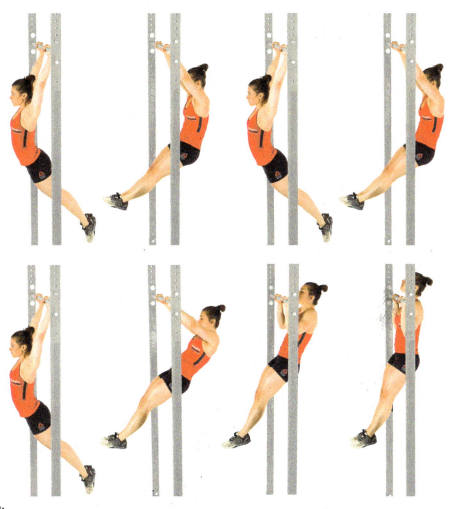

STEP 3:
- Two kip swings and a pull-up.

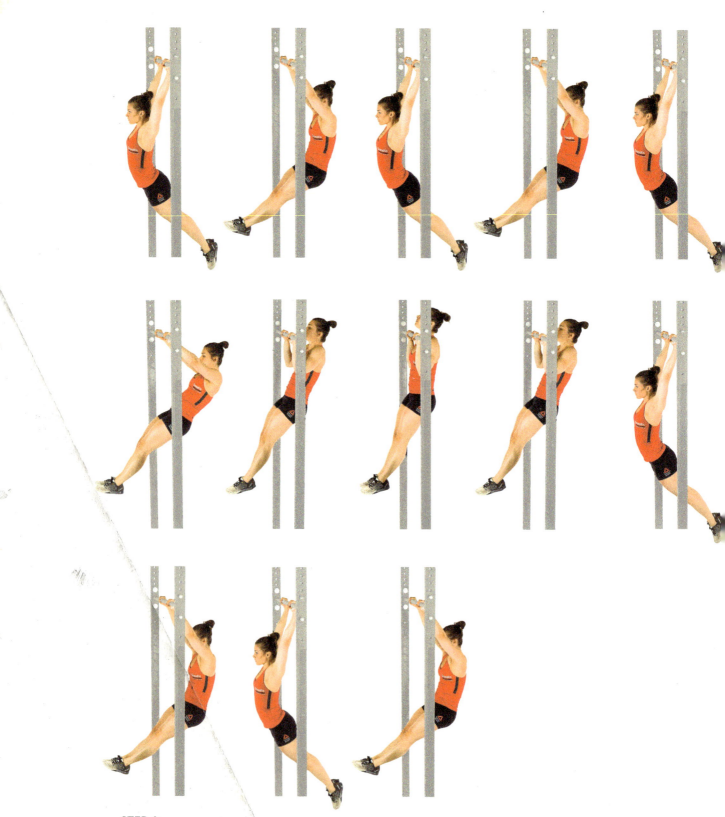

STEP 4:
- Two kip swings, a pull-up, and two kip swings.

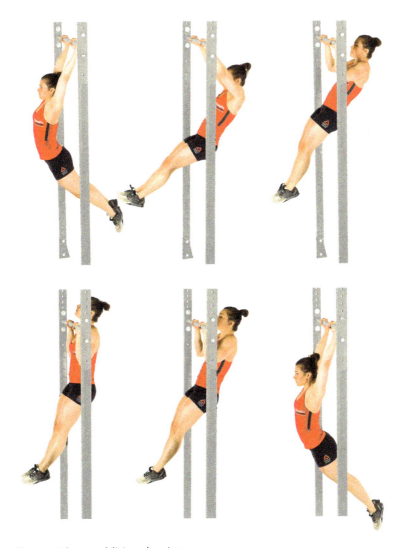

STEP 5:
- Multiple pull-ups without additional swings.

THE PULL-UP COMMON FAULTS AND CORRECTIONS

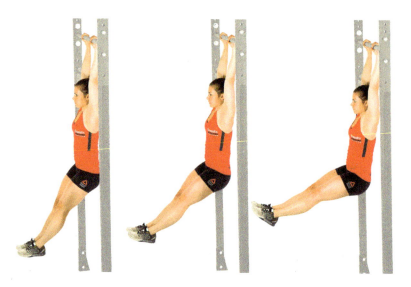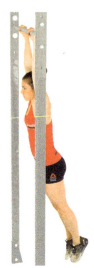

FAULT:

- Initiating the swing with the legs.

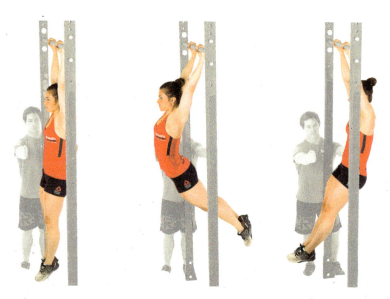

CORRECTION:

- Have the athlete go back in the progression to the kip swing and initiate the movement from the shoulders.

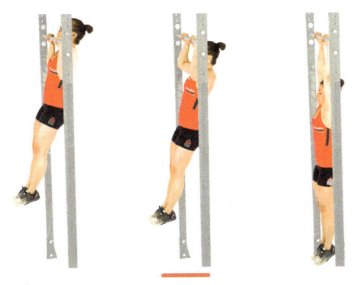

FAULT:

- Not pushing away after clearing the bar, sending the athlete straight down instead of following the arc of the kip swing.

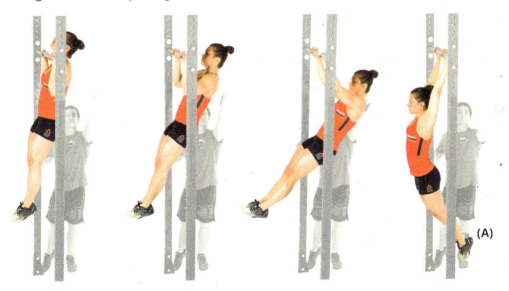

(A)

CORRECTIONS:

- Have the athlete pause at the top of the pull-up, focusing on pushing away from the bar.
- Have the athlete perform two kip swings in between each pull-up, practicing a sound return.
- Give the athlete a target at the back to encourage him or her to push away. **(A)**

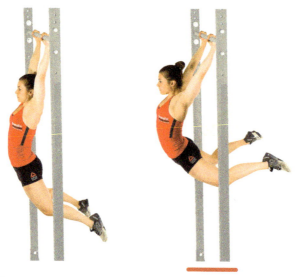

FAULT:

- Losing midline stabilization by overextending the spine or exaggerating the swing.

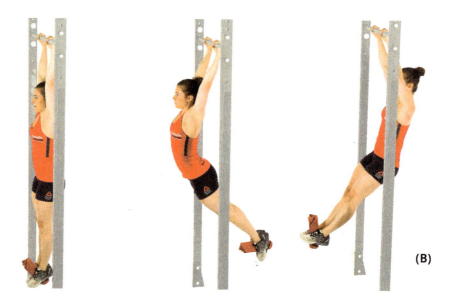

(B)

CORRECTIONS:

- Have the athlete work on the kip swing in a tighter position by keeping the legs together and the knees straight.
- Have the athlete put a towel between his or her feet to encourage a tight body position. **(B)**

THE THRUSTER

The thruster combines the front squat and push press in a single movement. Unlike the loose fingertip grip used in the front squat, the thruster requires a full grip on the bar and a lower elbow position. The athlete must move in a core-to-extremity movement pattern by extending the hip then pressing.

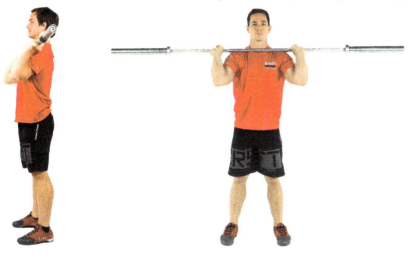

1. SET-UP

- Elbows in front of the bar.
- Bar rests on front rack.
- Hands just outside shoulders.
- Full grip on the bar.
- Shoulder-width stance.

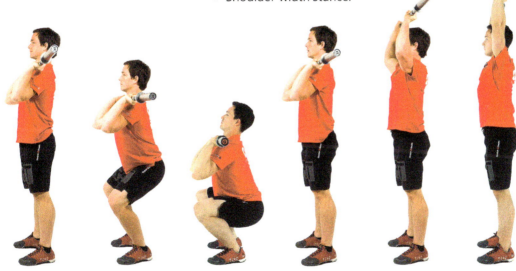

2. EXECUTION

- Hips descend back and down.
- Hips descend lower than knees.
- Lumbar curve maintained.
- Knees in line with toes.
- Elbows stay off knees.
- Hips and knees extend rapidly, then arms press.
- Heels down until hips and knees extend.
- Bar moves over the middle of the foot.

3. FINISH

- Complete at full hip, knee and arm extension.

THE THRUSTER TEACHING PROGRESSION

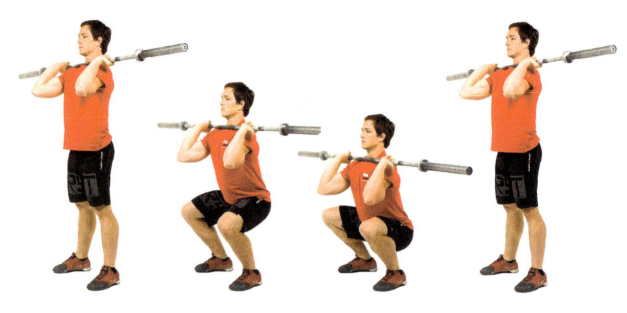

STEP 1:

- Front squat.

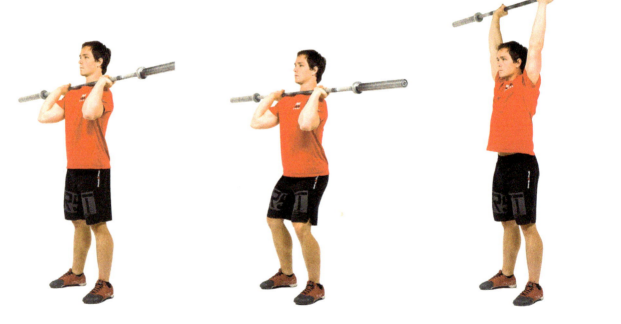

STEP 2:

- Push press (wide stance).

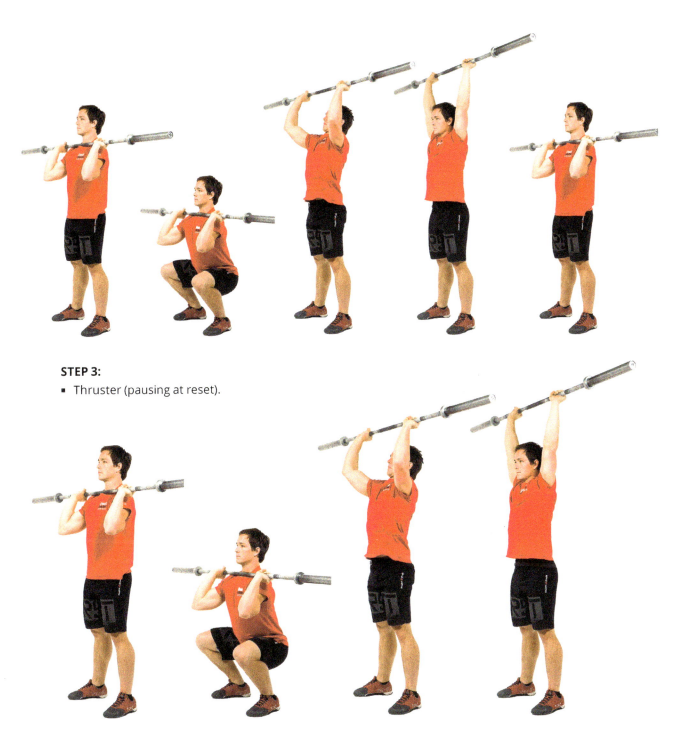

STEP 3:

- Thruster (pausing at reset).

STEP 4:

- Multiple thrusters (no pausing at any point in the movement).

THE THRUSTER COMMON FAULTS AND CORRECTIONS

Most faults and fixes from the front squat and push press apply to this movement, plus the following:

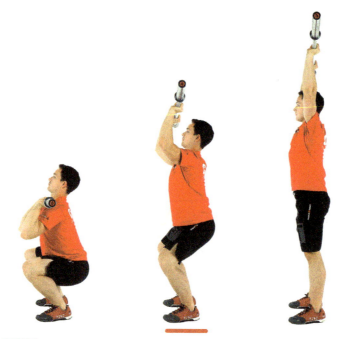

FAULT:

- Pressing the bar before extending the hips.

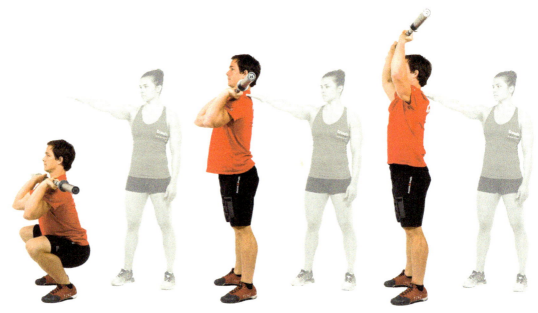

CORRECTION:

- Use a tactile cue and instruct the athlete to hit the hand before pressing.

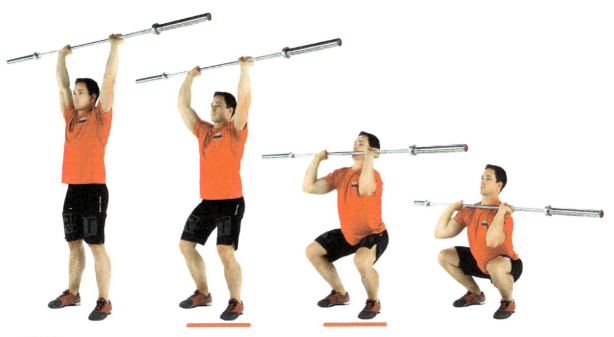

FAULT:
- Descending into the squat before the bar is in the rack position.

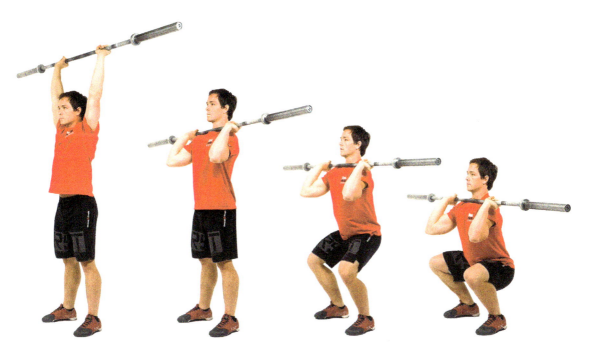

CORRECTION:
- Take the athlete back in the progression and have him or her pause at the rack position before squatting.

THE MUSCLE-UP

The muscle-up combines the pull-up and dip into one movement. The athlete pulls from a hang to a position of support, in this case above the rings. The false grip and the positioning of the rings during the transition are the keys to linking the pull-up and dip. Due to the dynamic nature of the rings, CrossFit recommends athletes achieve a strict muscle-up before attempting kipping muscle-ups.

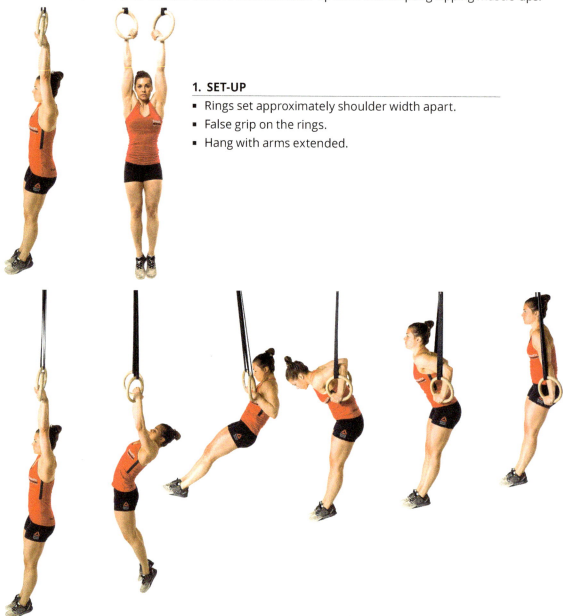

1. SET-UP

- Rings set approximately shoulder width apart.
- False grip on the rings.
- Hang with arms extended.

2. EXECUTION

- Pull rings to sternum as torso leans back.
- Move the chest over the rings; hands and elbows stay close to body.

3. FINISH

- Complete at full arm extension in support position.

THE MUSCLE-UP TEACHING PROGRESSION

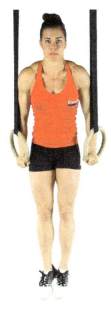

STEP 1:
- Ring support.

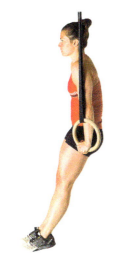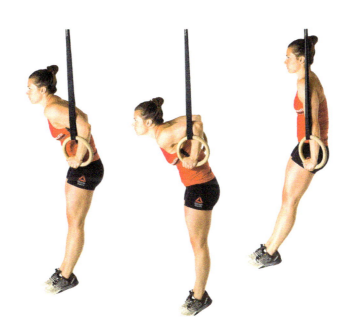

STEP 2:
- Ring dip.

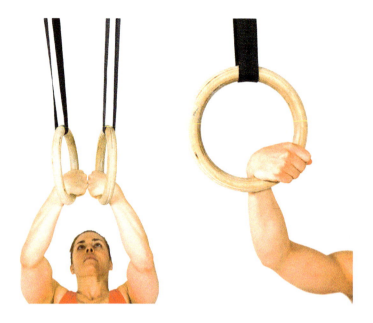

STEP 3:

- False grip.

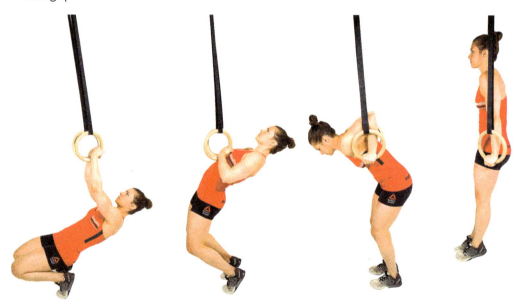

STEP 4:

- Kneeling muscle-ups. Raise the rings or move the feet further in front of the athlete to increase the challenge.

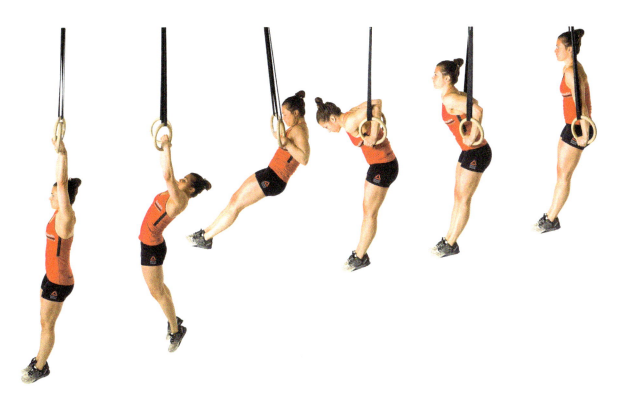

STEP 5
- Muscle-up.

THE MUSCLE-UP COMMON FAULTS AND CORRECTIONS

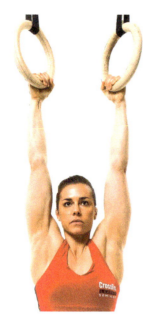
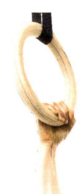
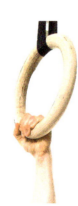

FAULT:
- Losing the false grip.

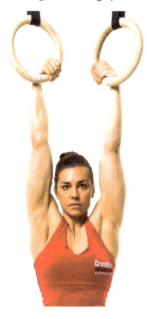
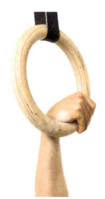
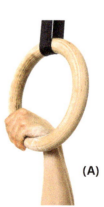

(A)

CORRECTIONS:
- Ensure the false grip is set before beginning a repetition. **(A)**
- Allow the athlete to use bent arms as he or she continues to develop the strength to hold the false grip with extended elbows.

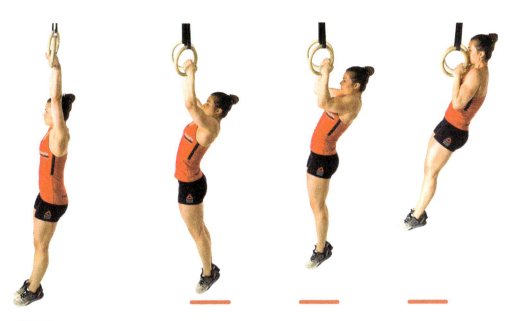

FAULT:

- Keeping the body too vertical in the pull so that the rings will not be in a position for an efficient transition.

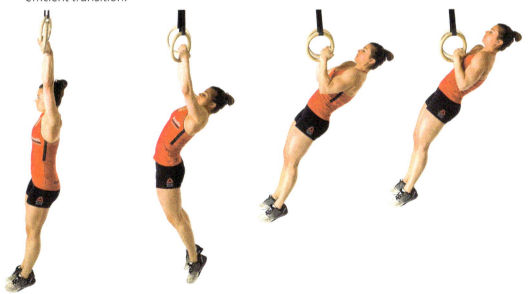

CORRECTION:

- Lean back so the rings can be pulled to the chest.

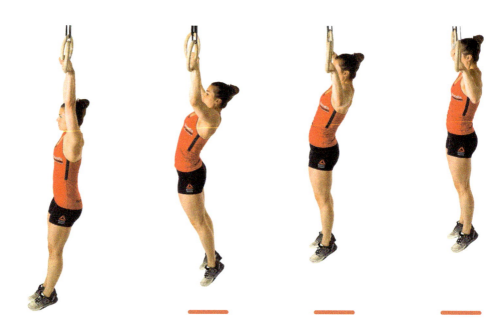

FAULT:

- Letting the elbows flare during the pull or transition.

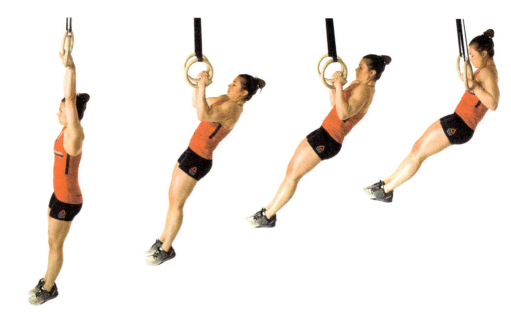

CORRECTION:

- Have the athlete keep the elbows close to the ribcage throughout the movement.

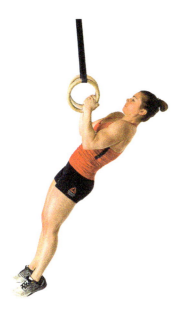

FAULT:
- Not pulling the rings low enough before beginning the transition.

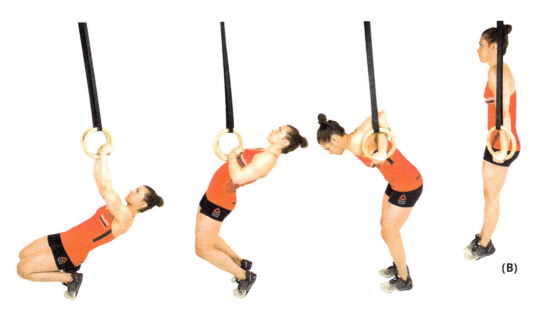

(B)

CORRECTIONS:
- Cue the athlete to lean back and pull the rings to the sternum before beginning the transition.
- Have the athlete go back in the progression to the kneeling muscle-up drill, selecting a ring height that is challenging. **(B)**

THE SNATCH

The snatch—the world's fastest lift—moves the barbell from the ground to overhead in one movement. Its complexity brings great benefit to CrossFit athletes.

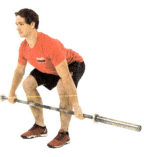

1. SET-UP

- Hip-width stance.
- Hands wide enough that bar rests in crease of hips when knees and hips are extended.
- Hook grip on the bar.
- Shoulders slightly in front of the bar.
- Eyes on the horizon.

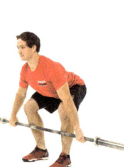
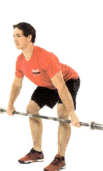
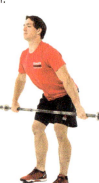
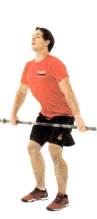

2. EXECUTION

- Lumbar curve maintained.
- Hips and shoulders rise at the same rate.
- Hips then extend rapidly.

- Heels down until hips and knees extend.
- Shoulders shrug, followed by a pull-under with the arms.

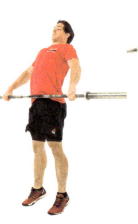
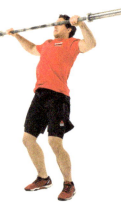
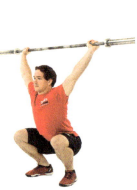
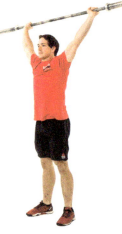

EXECUTION, CONTINUED

- Bar is received at the bottom of an overhead squat.

3. FINISH

- Complete at full hip, knee and arm extension with the bar over the middle of the foot.

THE SNATCH TEACHING PROGRESSION

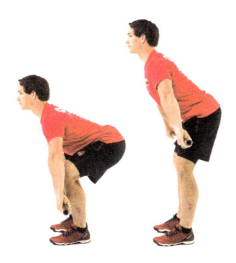

STEP 1:

- Deadlift to mid-thigh.

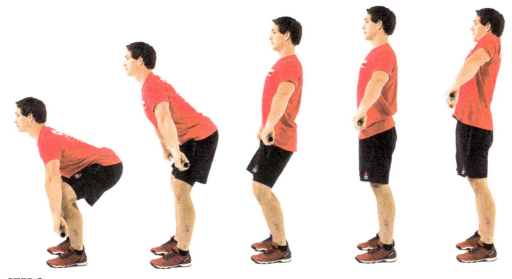

STEP 2:

- Deadlift-shrug.

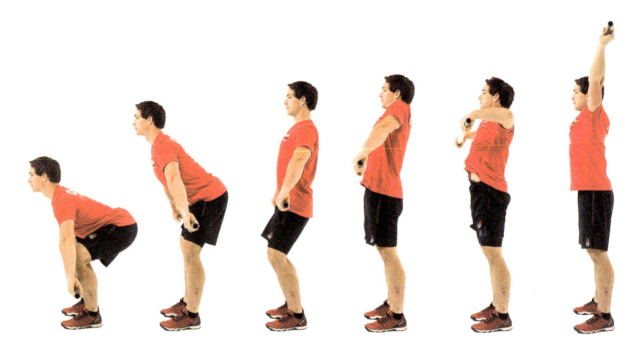

STEP 3:

- Muscle snatch.

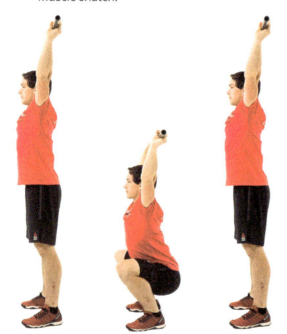

STEP 4:

- Overhead squat.

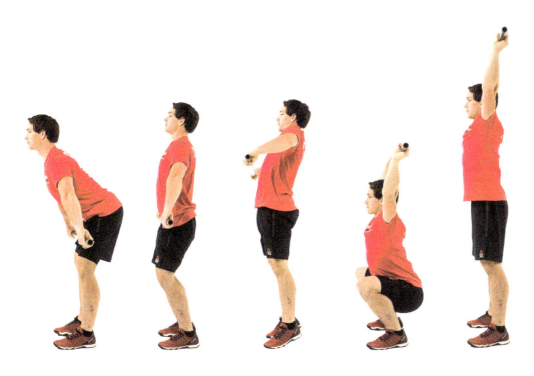

STEP 5:

- Hang snatch.

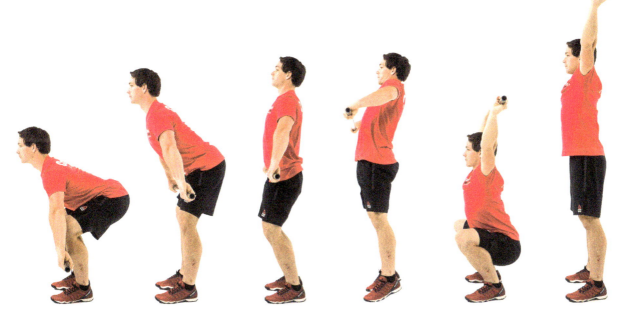

STEP 6:

- Snatch.

THE SNATCH COMMON FAULTS AND CORRECTIONS

Most faults and fixes from the deadlift, sumo deadlift high pull, and medicine-ball clean apply to this movement, plus the following:

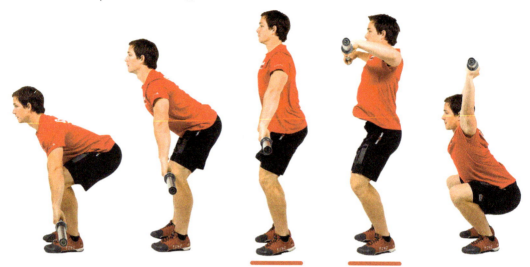

FAULT:

- Lack of hip extension.

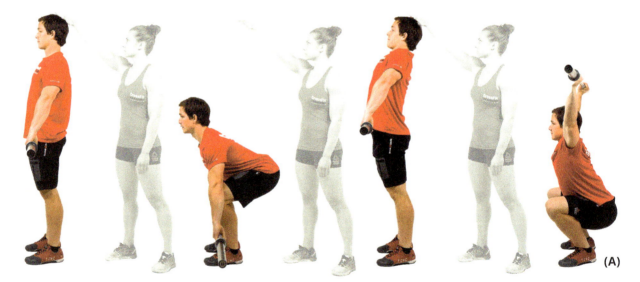

(A)

CORRECTIONS:

- Cue "Jump higher!"
- Place your hand at the top of the athlete's head when he or she is fully standing; keep it at that height and then ask the athlete to hit your hand during the drive. **(A)**
- Have the athlete perform two snatch deadlift-shrugs for every one snatch.

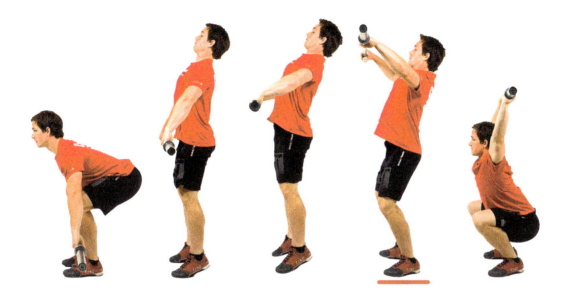

FAULT:

- Not moving the elbows high and outside or moving the bar around the body.

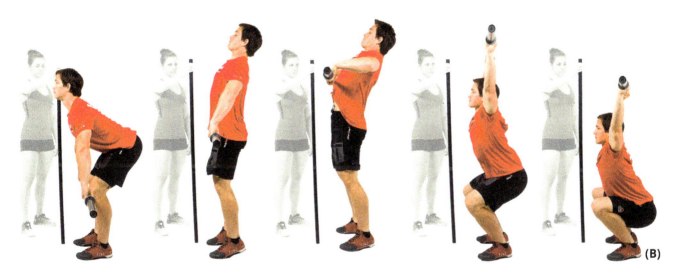

(B)

CORRECTIONS:

- If the athlete is using PVC, use a tactile cue to prevent him or her from swinging the bar out in front. **(B)**
- Cue "Elbows high and outside!"
- Cue the athlete to brush his or her shirt with the PVC/barbell.

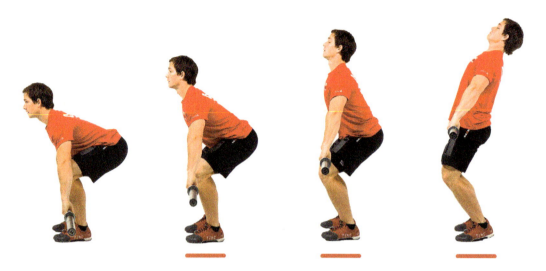

FAULT:

- Shoulders rise without the hips.

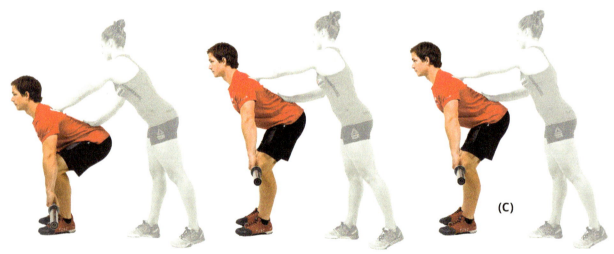

(C)

CORRECTIONS:

- Cue "Push the knees back as your chest rises."
- Be sure the athlete is set up correctly and the hips are not too low.
- Give a tactile cue at the hips and shoulders to have them lift in unison. **(C)**

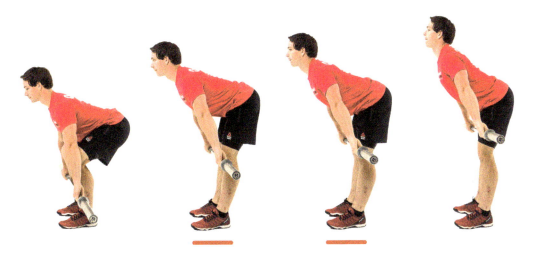

FAULT:

- Hips rise without the shoulders.

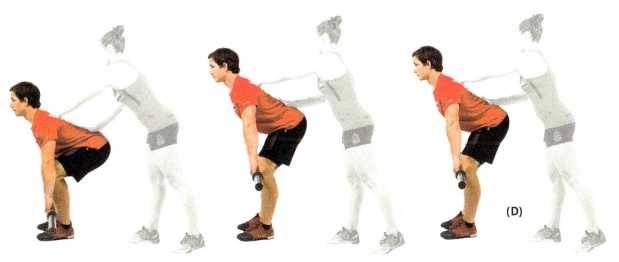

(D)

CORRECTIONS:

- Cue "Keep the chest lifted as you straighten your legs."
- Be sure the athlete is set up correctly and the hips are not too high.
- Give a tactile cue at the hips and shoulders to have them lift in unison. **(D)**

INDEX

ALPHABETICAL LISTING OF FIGURES

ALPHABETICAL LISTING OF TABLES